W0018983

THE *MORE* DANGEROUS CASE OF DONALD TRUMP

40 PSYCHIATRISTS AND MENTAL HEALTH EXPERTS WARN ANEW

Edited by

Bandy X. Lee, M.D., M.Div.

World Mental Health Coalition, Inc.

New York

A World Mental Health Coalition Book

The More Dangerous Case of Donald Trump:
40 Psychiatrists and Mental Health Experts Warn Anew
Copyright © 2024 by Bandy X. Lee, M.D., M.Div.
All rights reserved. Printed in the United States of America.

www.worldmhc.org
www.bandylee.com

Cover design Stacey L. Pritchett
Special consultant Prudence Gourguechon, M.D.
Editorial assistant Gloria Schroeter

Library of Congress Cataloging-in-Publication Data available upon request.

ISBN 979-8-9900533-7-3 (softcover)
ISBN 979-8-9900533-6-6 (ebook)

This work is dedicated to the American people,
whom we serve.

CONTENTS

FOREWORD TO THE FIRST EDITION
Our Witness to Malignant Normality
ROBERT JAY LIFTON, M.D.

(This is a lightly edited excerpt of the original Foreword for The Dangerous Case of Donald Trump: 27 Psychiatrists and Mental Health Experts Assess a President.*)*

Our situation as American psychological professionals can be summed up in just two ideas—we can call them themes or even concepts: First, what I call *malignant normality*, which has to do with the social actuality with which we are presented as normal, all-encompassing, and unalterable; and second, our potential and crucial sense of ourselves as *witnessing professionals*.

Concerning malignant normality, we start with an assumption that all societies, at various levels of consciousness, put forward ways of viewing, thinking, and behaving that are considered desirable or "normal." Yet, these criteria for normality can be much affected by the political and military currents of a particular era. Such requirements may be fairly benign, but they can also be destructive to the point of evil.

I came to the idea of malignant normality in my study of Nazi doctors. Those assigned to Auschwitz, when taking charge of the selections and the overall killing process, were simply doing what was expected of them. True, some were upset, even horrified, at being given this task. Yet, with a certain amount of counseling—one can call it perverse psychotherapy—offered by more experienced hands, a process that included drinking heavily together and giving assurance of help and support, the great majority could overcome their anxiety sufficiently to carry through their murderous assignment. This was a process of *adaptation to evil* that is all too possible to initiate in such a situation. Above all, there was a *normalization of evil* that enhanced this adaption and served to present

I

participating doctors with the Auschwitz institution as the existing world to which one must make one's adjustments.

There is another form of malignant normality closer to home and more recent. I have in mind the participation in torture by physicians (including psychiatrists), and by psychologists, and other medical and psychological personnel. This reached its most extreme manifestation when two psychologists were revealed to be among architects of the CIA's torture protocol. More than that, this malignant normality was essentially supported by the American Psychological Association in its defense of the participation of psychologists in the so-called "enhanced interrogation" techniques that spilled over into torture.

I am not equating this American behavior with the Nazi example, but rather suggesting that malignant normality can take different forms. And nothing does more to sustain malignant normality than its support from a large organization of professionals.

There is still another kind of malignant normality, one brought about by [former] President Trump and his administration. Judith Herman and I, in a letter to the New York Times in March 2017, stressed Trump's dangerous individual psychological patterns: his creation of his own reality, and his inability to manage the inevitable crises that face an American president. He has also, in various ways, violated our American institutional requirements and threatened the viability of American democracy. A dangerous president becomes normalized, and malignant normality comes to dominate our governing (or, one could say our anti-governing) dynamic. But that does not mean we are helpless. Unlike Nazi doctors, articulate psychological professionals could and did expose the behavior of corrupt colleagues and even a corrupt professional society. Investigative journalists and human rights groups also greatly contributed to that exposure.

This brings me to my second theme, that of witnessing professionals, particularly activist witnessing professionals. Most professionals, most of the time, operate within the norms (that is, the criteria for normality) of their particular society. Indeed, professionals often go further, and in their practices may deepen the commitment of people they work with to that normality. This can give solace, but it has its perils.

It is not generally known that during the early Cold War period, a special governmental commission, chaired by a psychiatrist and containing physicians and social scientists, was set up to help the American people achieve the desired psychological capacity to support U.S. stockpiling of nuclear weapons; cope with an anticipated nuclear attack and overcome the fear of nuclear annihilation. The commission had the task, in short, of helping Americans accept malignant nuclear normality. There have also been parallel examples in recent history of professionals who have promoted equally dangerous forms of normality in rejecting climate change.

But professionals don't have to serve these forms of malignant normality. We are capable of using our knowledge and technical skills to expose such normality, to bear witness to its malignance, to become witnessing professionals.

When I did my study of Hiroshima survivors back in 1962, I sought to uncover, in the most accurate and scientific way I could, the psychological and bodily experience of people exposed to the atomic bomb. Yet, I was not just a neutral observer. Over time, I came to understand myself as a witnessing professional, committed to making known what an atomic bomb could do to a city, to tell the world something of what had happened in Hiroshima and to its inhabitants. For me Hiroshima meant "one plane, one bomb, one city." I came to view this commitment to telling Hiroshima's story as a form of advocacy research. That meant combining a disciplined professional approach with the ethical requirements of committed witness, combining scholarship with activism.

I believe that some such approach is what we require now, in the Trump era. We need to avoid uncritical acceptance of this new version of malignant normality and, instead, bring our knowledge and experience to exposing it for what it is. This requires us to be disciplined about what we believe we know, while refraining from holding forth on what we do not know. It also requires us to recognize the urgency of the situation in which the most powerful man in the world is also the bearer of profound instability and untruth. As psychological professionals, we act with ethical passion in our efforts to reveal what is most dangerous and what, in contrast, might be life-affirming in the face of the malignant normality that surrounds us.

Finally, there is the issue of our ethical behavior. We talk a lot about our professional ethics having to do with our responsibility to patients and to the overall standards of our discipline. This concern with professional ethics matters a great deal.

But I am suggesting something more—a larger concept of professional ethics that we don't often discuss, including whom we work for and with, and how our work either affirms or questions the directions of the larger society. And in our present situation, how we deal with the malignant normality that faces us.

I in no way minimize the significance of professional knowledge and technical skill. But our professions can become overly technicized, too much like hired guns able to bring their firepower to any sponsor of the most egregious view of normality.

III

We can do better than that. We can take the larger ethical view of the activist witnessing professional. Bandy Lee took that view when organizing the Yale conference, and the participants affirmed it. This does not make us saviors of our threatened society. But it does help us bring our experience and knowledge to bear on what threatens us and what might renew us.

A line from the American poet, Theodore Roethke brings eloquence to what I have been trying to say:

In a dark time, the eye begins to see.

Robert Jay Lifton, M.D., is Lecturer in Psychiatry at Columbia University and Distinguished Professor Emeritus of John Jay College and the Graduate Center of the City University of New York. A leading psychohistorian, he studied Hiroshima survivors and the doctors who aided Nazi war crimes. He was an outspoken critic of the American Psychological Association's aiding of government-sanctioned torture, and is a vocal opponent of nuclear weapons. His most recent books are Losing Reality: On Cults, Cultism, and the Mindset of Political and Religious Zealotry, and Surviving Our Catastrophes: Resilience and Renewal from Hiroshima to the COVID-19 Pandemic.

PROLOGUE TO THE FIRST EDITION
Professions and Politics
Judith Lewis Herman, M.D., and Bandy X. Lee, M.D., M.Div.

(This is a lightly edited excerpt of the original Prologue for The Dangerous Case of Donald Trump: 27 Psychiatrists and Mental Health Experts Assess a President.*)*

Professions can create forms of ethical conversation that are impossible between a lonely individual and a distant government. If members of professions think of themselves as groups … with norms and rules that oblige them at all times, then they can gain … confidence, and indeed a certain kind of power.

Timothy Snyder, *On Tyranny:*
Twenty Lessons from the Twentieth Century (2017)

Norms and rules guide professional conduct, set standards, and point to the essential principles of practice. For these reasons, physicians have the *Declaration of Geneva* (World Medical Association, 2006) and the American Medical Association (AMA) *Principles of Medical Ethics* (AMA, 2001), which guide the APA's code for psychiatry (APA, 2013). The former confirms the physician's dedication to the humanitarian goals of medicine, while the latter defines honorable behavior for the physician. Paramount in both is the health, safety, and survival of the patient.

If we are mindful of the dangers of politicizing the professions, then certainly we must heed the so-called "Goldwater rule," or Section 7.3 of the APA code of ethics, which states:

It is unethical for a psychiatrist to offer a professional opinion [on a public figure] unless he or she has conducted an examination and has been granted proper authorization for such a statement (APA, 2013). This is not divergent from ordinary norms of practice; the clinical approaches that we use to evaluate patients require a full examination. Formulating a credible diagnosis will always be limited when applied to public figures observed outside this intimate frame; in fact, we would go so far as to assert that it is impossible.

However, the public trust is also violated if the profession fails in its duty to alert the public when a person who holds the power of life and death over us all shows signs of clear, dangerous mental impairment. We should pause if professionals are asked to remain silent when they have seen enough evidence to sound alarm in every other situation. In a democracy, should not the president, as First Citizen, be subject to the same standards of practice as the rest of the citizenry when it comes to dangerousness?

The physician, to whom life-and-death situations are entrusted, is expected to know when it is appropriate to act, and to act responsibly when warranted. It is because of the weight of this responsibility that, rightfully, the physician should refrain from commenting on a public figure except in the rarest instance. Only in an emergency should a physician breach the trust of confidentiality and intervene without consent, and only in an emergency should a physician breach the Goldwater rule. We believe that such an emergency now exists.

Test for Proper Responsibility

We are asking our fellow mental health professionals to get involved in politics not only as citizens (a right most of us still enjoy), but also, specifically, as professionals and as guardians of special knowledge with which they have been entrusted. How can we be sure that this is permissible? It is all too easy to claim, just as we have done, that an emergency situation requires a departure from our usual practices in the private sphere. How can we judge whether in fact our political involvement is justified?

We would argue that the key question is whether professionals are engaging in political *collusion* with state abuses of power, or in *resistance* to them. If we are asked to cooperate with state programs that violate human rights, then regardless of the purported justification, any involvement can only corrupt, and the only appropriate ethical stance is to refuse participation of any sort. If, on the other hand, we perceive that state power is being abused by an executive who seems to be mentally unstable, then we may certainly speak out, not only as citizens, but also, we would argue, as professionals who are privy to special information and a responsibility to educate the public. For whatever our wisdom and expertise may be worth, surely, we are obligated to share it.

It doesn't take a psychiatrist to notice that our president is mentally compromised. Nevertheless, by speaking out as professionals, we lend support and dignity to our fellow citizens who are justifiably alarmed by the president's furious tirades, conspiracy fantasies, aversion to facts, and attraction to violence. We can lend a hand in helping the public to understand behaviors that are unusual and alarming, which can all too easily be rationalized and normalized.

A man can be both evil and mentally compromised—which is a more frightening proposition. Power not only corrupts, but also magnifies existing psychopathologies, even as it creates new ones. Fostered by the flattery of underlings and the chants of crowds, a political leader's grandiosity may morph into grotesque delusions of grandeur. Sociopathic traits may be amplified as the leader discovers that he can violate the norms of civil society and even commit crimes with impunity. And the leader who rules through fear, lies, and betrayal may become increasingly isolated and paranoid, as the loyalty of even his closest confidants must forever be suspect.

Some would argue that by paying attention to the [former] president's mental state, we are colluding with him in deflecting attention from his actions, upon which he should ultimately be judged (Frances, 2017). Certainly, mental disturbance is not an excuse for tyrannical behavior; nevertheless, it cannot be ignored. In a court of law, even the strongest insanity defense case cannot show that a person is insane all the time. We submit that by paying attention to the [former] president's mental state *as well as* his actions, we are better informed to assess his dangerousness.

Delusional levels of grandiosity, impulsivity, and compulsions of mental impairment, when combined with an authoritarian cult of personality and contempt for the rule of law, are a toxic mix. We collectively warn that anyone as mentally unstable as this man simply should not be entrusted with the life-and-death powers of the presidency.

Judith Lewis Herman, M.D., is Senior Lecturer in Psychiatry at Harvard Medical School. She is a renowned expert in the traumas of interpersonal violence and author of the now classic Trauma and Recovery: The Aftermath of Violence—from Domestic Abuse to Political Terror. *She is a Distinguished Life Fellow of the American Psychiatric Association and the recipient of numerous awards, including the Lifetime Achievement Award from International Society for Traumatic Stress Studies. Her most recent book,* Truth and Repair: How Trauma Survivors Envision Justice, *was published in 2023.*

Bandy X. Lee, M.D., M.Div., is a forensic and social psychiatrist who taught at Yale School of Medicine and Yale Law School for 17 years before joining the Harvard Program in Psychiatry and the Law. She edited The Dangerous Case of Donald Trump: 27 Psychiatrists and Mental Health Experts Assess a President, *in order to warn the public of a national public health emergency. She is President of the World Mental Health Coalition and Cofounder of the Violence Prevention Institute. She most recently authored* The Psychology of Trump Contagion: An Existential Danger to American Democracy and All Humankind.

References

American Medical Association (2001). *AMA Code of Medical Ethics: AMA Principles of Medical Ethics*. Chicago, IL: American Medical Association. Retrieved from https://www.ama-assn.org/sites/default/files/media-browser/principles-of-medical-ethics.pdf

American Psychiatric Association (2013). *Principles of Medical Ethics with Annotations Especially Applicable to Psychiatry*. Arlington, VA: American Psychiatric Association. Retrieved from https://www.psychiatry.org/psychiatrists/practice/ethics

Frances, A. (2017, February 14). An eminent psychiatrist demurs on Trump's mental state. *New York Times*. Retrieved from https://www.nytimes.com/2017/02/14/opinion/an-eminent-psychiatrist-demurs-on-trumps-mental-state.html

Snyder, T. (2017). *On Tyranny: Twenty Lessons from the Twentieth Century.* New York, NY: Crown/Archetype

World Medical Association (2006). *Declaration of Geneva*. Geneva, Switzerland: World Medical Association. Retrieved from https://www.wma.net/policies-post/wma-declaration-of-geneva/

PROLOGUE TO THE SECOND EDITION
Professions and Activism
STEPHEN SOLDZ, PH.D., AND BANDY X. LEE, M.D., M.DIV.

(This is a lightly edited excerpt of the original Prologue for The Dangerous Case of Donald Trump: 37 Psychiatrists and Mental Health Experts Assess a President.*)*

Professionals are an important component in helping to provide checks on powerful institutions and alerting the public to wrongs. Professions operate with an implicit social contract with the broader society to contribute their special knowledge and training to the greater good. Their member professionals agree to follow a professional ethics code that binds them beyond the ordinary citizen. In exchange, these professionals are granted certain privileges not available to all in the wider society. For example, lawyers are expected to act in the best interests of their clients and to adhere to attorney-client privilege.

Health professionals pledge to use their knowledge and expertise to improve people's lives and "to do no harm." At times they must sacrifice their comfort and even family commitments to attend to their patients' needs. They also pledge to keep the confidences their patients communicate to them. In exchange, physicians and psychologists, among other professionals, are granted privileges such as an inviolable confidentiality of those communications, often even from law enforcement or the courts. In war, doctors are given such special status under the Geneva Conventions that the First Geneva Convention stipulates that:

Medical personnel exclusively engaged in the search for, or the collection, transport or treatment of the wounded or sick, or in the prevention of disease, staff exclusively engaged in the administration of medical units and establishments…

IX

shall be respected and protected in all circumstances (International Committee of the Red Cross, 2016).

These principles are incorporated into the World Medical Association's Physician's Pledge of the Declaration of Geneva, developed in the wake of World War II, which some consider to be the modern-day Hippocratic Oath. The most relevant clauses from the Declaration are:

AS A MEMBER OF THE MEDICAL PROFESSION:

I SOLEMNLY PLEDGE to dedicate my life to the service of humanity;

THE HEALTH AND WELL-BEING OF MY PATIENT will be my first consideration;

I WILL RESPECT the autonomy and dignity of my patient;

I WILL MAINTAIN the utmost respect for human life;

I WILL NOT PERMIT considerations of age, disease or disability, creed, ethnic origin, gender, nationality, political affiliation, race, sexual orientation, social standing or any other factor to intervene between my duty and my patient;
....
I WILL NOT USE my medical knowledge to violate human rights and civil liberties, even under threat (World Medical Association, 2017).

Despite minor differences, all medical professions share certain foundational ethical principles embodied in the Physician's Pledge. Among these are *beneficence, nonmaleficence, justice,* and respect for the *autonomy* of individuals. Beneficence refers to the obligation that health professionals are supposed to use their knowledge and expertise for the benefit of people, including both their patients and the wider public. Nonmaleficence refers to the famous "do no harm" clause and is often considered to be the first principle of healthcare, as in "first, do no harm." Thus, when consistent with beneficence, we health professionals should not apply ineffective or harmful treatments. This obligation also applies to the wider society, obligating us to take steps to prevent an infectious patient from infecting others, even if those others are not our patients.

Dr. Soldz spent a decade working to expose the roles of psychologists and other health professionals in the government's torture program and to change Association's policies to be more consistent with those of the medical and psychiatric associations. On the one hand, as a citizen-professional concerned about the spread of brutality in our society, he acted on his outrage as a health professional that our government was resorting to officially authorized torture. While the United States has had a long and disturbing relationship with torture,(Marks 1991; McCoy 2006, 2012; Otterman 2007) it seemed a major step toward the brutalization of society to adopt torture as official policy.(Cole 2009) This official acceptance of torture could lead to acceptance of other forms of brutalization, both in other countries and against people in the United States. While acting as a citizen, he was simultaneously acting as a professional psychologist concerned that participation in torture was undermining the ethical basis of his profession. As a result of the actions of Dr. Soldz and other dozens of activists over many years, the Association changed its policies after Hoffman filed his report in 2015 (Aldhous 2015; Welch 2009).

Dr. Lee, who has devoted her life to the study and prevention of violence, has argued forcefully that social, cultural, economic, and environmental factors are far more reliable predictors of violence than individual factors (Lee 2018). Based on this experience, after [Donald] Trump's election, she became concerned that the public health effects of having a psychologically unstable president would be highly consequential and widespread. Subsequent events unfortunately have shown only too clearly that her fears were well founded, as we have seen thousands of children separated from their migrant families in ways that may have permanently traumatized them; cruel hardships created for the 40 million Americans living in poverty in perhaps the greatest wealth transfer from the poor to the wealthy in U.S. history; white supremacist killings doubling while gun murder rates have escalated to levels not seen in 25 years; encouragement of violence against journalists while excusing the murder of journalists abroad; reversal of the small steps that the U.S. has taken to reduce the threats from global warming; [the U.S. becoming the global epicenter of Covid-19 deaths from pandemic mismanagement; the U.S. falling from its status as the longest continuous democracy, after a violent insurrection against the government;] and a restructuring of the geopolitical order that has emboldened dictators, reignited a nuclear arms race, and generated a hostile political environment, both at home and abroad.

Now that the psychological dangerousness of Donald Trump has translated into geopolitical dangerousness and the dangers have vastly increased, the American Psychiatric Association, sadly, has become an epitome of institutional complicity and betrayal (Smith and Freyd, 2014) and another example of how an organization charged with establishing ethical guidelines has rather become an agent of the state. We must remember that the Declaration of Geneva Physician's Pledge was adopted in 1948 as a clarification of the health professional's humanitarian obligation, after the experience of Nazism, that *either* silence *or* active cooperation on the part of professionals with a dangerous regime could contribute to atrocities.

These varied experiences illustrate that there comes a point where mental health and other health professionals' professional roles and their roles as citizens begin to merge. There is also tension among professionals regarding how to act as purveyors of ideas and as doers. We believe that our professional training teaches us to separate these roles so that we can merge them thoughtfully: there comes a point where ideas alone are insufficient for bringing the world to health and safety, and action without careful thought becomes dangerous for its potential to contribute to unintended results. These are healthy tensions that will likely never receive a final resolution but will have to be renegotiated generation by generation and struggle by struggle. It is our hope that the contributions to the present book will help our generation explore these tensions we mental health professionals experience as we join with fellow citizens in efforts to do our part in healing and coping with the dangerous territory facing our country and the world.

Stephen Soldz, Ph.D., is a clinical psychologist and psychoanalyst in Boston. He is Professor at the Boston Graduate School of Psychoanalysis. Over the past two decades he was a leader in efforts to end U.S. torture and to remove psychologists from participation in abusive interrogations and other problematic military and intelligence operations. Soldz is President-Elect of the Society for Psychoanalysis and Psychoanalytic Psychology (Division 39 of the American Psychological Association), past President of Psychologists for Social Responsibility, a Cofounder of the Coalition for an Ethical Psychology, and an Anti-Torture Adviser for Physicians for Human Rights.

Bandy X. Lee, M.D., M.Div., is a forensic and social psychiatrist who taught at Yale School of Medicine and Yale Law School for 17 years before joining the Harvard Program in Psychiatry and the Law. She edited The Dangerous Case of Donald Trump: 27 Psychiatrists and Mental Health Experts Assess a President, *in order to warn the public of a national public health emergency. She is President of the World Mental Health Coalition and Cofounder of the Violence Prevention Institute. She most recently authored* The Psychology of Trump Contagion: An Existential Danger to American Democracy and All Humankind.

References

Aldhous, P. (2015, August 7). How six rebel psychologists fought a decade-long war on torture—and won. *Buzzfeed.* Retrieved from https://www.buzzfeednews.com/article/peteraldhous/the-dissidents?

Cole, D. (2009). *The Torture Memos: Rationalizing the Unthinkable.* New York, NY: New Press.

International Committee of the Red Cross (2016). Treaties, states, parties, and commentaries—Geneva Convention (I) on wounded and sick in Armed Forces in the field. 1949—24—Article 24: Protection of permanent personnel—commentary of 2016. Retrieved from https://ihl-databases.icrc.org/applic/ihl/ihl.nsf/Comment.xsp?action=openDocument&documentId=8BB42A7717B581D5C1257F15004A199F

Lee, B. (2018, March 6). Violence is a societal disorder. *US News & World Report.* Retrieved from https://www.usnews.com/opinion/policy-dose/articles/2018-03-06/prevent-violence-at-the-societal-level

Marks, J. D. (1991). *The Search for the 'Manchurian Candidate.'* New York, NY: Norton.

McCoy, A. W. (2006). *A Question of Torture: CIA Interrogation, from the Cold War to the War on Terror.* 1st ed. The American Empire Project. New York, NY: Metropolitan Books/Henry Holt and Co. Retrieved from http://www.loc.gov/catdir/enhancements/fy0625/2005051124-b.html   http://www.loc.gov/catdir/enhancements/fy0625/2005051124-d.html.

Smith, C. P., & Freyd, J. J. (2014). Institutional Betrayal. *American Psychologist* (pp. 575–87). 69 (6)

Welch, B. (2009, July 21). The American Psychological Association and torture: The day the tide turned. *Huffington Post*. Retrieved from http://www.huffingtonpost.com/bryant-welch/the-american-psychologica_b_242020.html

World Medical Association (2017). *WMA Declaration of Geneva*. Geneva, Switzerland: World Medical Association. Retrieved from https://www.wma.net/policies-post/wma-declaration-of-geneva/

CW01499667

INTRODUCTION
Our Duty to Humanity
BANDY X. LEE, M.D., M.DIV.

Much has happened since the publication of our first public-service book, *The Dangerous Case of Donald Trump: 27 Psychiatrists and Mental Health Experts Assess a President* (Lee, 2017), which was such an unprecedented *New York Times* bestseller of its kind, that it took one of the Big Five publishers five weeks of repeat printings to catch up with the demand. We learned much later that White House Chief of Staff General John Kelly consulted our book as an "owner's manual" for dealing with the dangers of Donald Trump (Green, 2022a; Green, 2022b), which may have played a role in preventing a nuclear war with North Korea! Even General Mark Milley, former chairman of the Joint Chiefs of Staff, who took exceptional steps to prevent nuclear war in the last days of the Trump presidency, was recently spotted (as of the time of this writing) to be holding a copy of the expanded edition, *The Dangerous Case of Donald Trump: 37 Psychiatrists and Mental Health Experts Assess a President* (Lee, 2019). Adding ten more expert authors, this second edition had warned that, without containment, the psychological dangers we warned against would grow worse, and eventually spread into social, cultural, geopolitical, and civic dangers.

This is exactly what came to pass. I was moved to supplement these warnings with my own books: *Profile of a Nation: Trump's Mind, America's Soul* (Lee, 2020), which predicted a violent insurrection following the 2020 presidential election—as well as "a presidency that will not end" for Donald Trump, regardless of election results. Then I wrote *The Psychology of Trump Contagion: An Existential Danger to American Democracy and All Humankind* (Lee, 2024), which attempts to illustrate how prolonged exposure to a severely-impaired, powerful public figure results in a contagion of symptoms across populations. They each extend lessons learned from "the dangerous case of

Donald Trump."

Now, this current volume on "the *more* dangerous case of Donald Trump" updates the previous two compendia. It is released in conjunction with a major, multidisciplinary conference in the National Press Club Ballroom on September 27, 2024, which follows a similar major conference the year before the 2020 presidential election (C-Span, 2019). The meaning of "more" is multiple: more severe symptoms; more new symptoms and perhaps syndromes; more patrons and pawns; more people and nations afflicted with "Trump Contagion"; and more institutions and establishments, either opportunistically or obsequiously, joining to facilitate the "Death Spiral" of his pathological drive.

There was such great enthusiasm for this publication, it was a struggle to keep to a reasonable number of mental health experts, and in consultation with my gracious editorial help and former vice president of the World Mental Health Coalition, Dr. Prudence Gourguechon, we managed to keep it to forty. The sections are named, much as in psychiatric tradition, after Greek gods: "Thanatos", "Eros", "Harpocrates", and "Aesculapius". "Thanatos" refers to the death drive Donald Trump brings by virtue of his mental pathology. "Eros" refers to a life impulse, or our fundamental desire for love, acceptance, and belonging, which may manifest as tribalism, persecution of outgroups, and conformity when disordered. "Harpocrates" (not Hippocrates) refers to the God of Silence, or the silencing of experts by the American Psychiatric Association that seemed to me more harmful than the mental health crisis itself (even when symptoms are severe, the situation is salvageable if there is *insight*, or the ability to recognize that something is wrong and to seek help; our public voice facilitates this insight). Finally, "Aesculapius" is the God of Healing, whose rod is the symbol of medicine—the snake-entwined staff—that specks every medical student's vision for the task before them: to act in a way that protects from harm; restores life; and contributes to the wonders of human flourishing. Indeed, medicine is both an enormous privilege and an awesome responsibility that the Ancients conceded as worthy of our personal sacrifice.

No elaboration is necessary on how much more dangerous the world has become since Donald Trump's ascent to the U.S. presidency (Armed Conflict Location and Event Data, 2024; Lindsey and Dahlman, 2024). Many agree that this volume is coming together at an extremely precarious, even cataclysmic, time (Economist, 2023). I am immensely grateful to all the contributors here who are lending their expert voices, at potentially great risk to their safety, reputation, and livelihood, to offer their knowledge in service to humanity. In times of authoritarianism, it can be a challenge to tell the truth, since the truth empowers the public. Nevertheless, it is ultimately society that we serve, and society that will save us all.

Bandy X. Lee, M.D., M.Div., is a forensic and social psychiatrist who taught at Yale School of Medicine and Yale Law School for 17 years before joining the Harvard Program in Psychiatry and the Law. She edited The Dangerous Case of Donald Trump: 27 Psychiatrists and Mental Health Experts Assess a President, *in order to warn the public of a national public health emergency. She most recently authored* The Psychology of Trump Contagion: An Existential Danger to American Democracy and All Humankind. *Her work is dedicated to Mirabelle and Blake and to their future.*

References

Armed Conflict Location and Event Data (2024). ACLED Conflict Index Results: July 2024. Armed Conflict Location and Event Data. https://acleddata.com/conflict-index/index-july-2024/

C-Span (2019, March 19). The Dangerous Case of Donald Trump: 27 Psychiatrists and Mental Health Experts Assess a President. Washington, DC: C-Span. Retrieved from https://www.c-span.org/video/?458919-1/the-dangerous-case-donald-trump.

Economist (2023, November 16). Donald Trump poses the biggest danger to the world in 2024. *Economist.* https://www.economist.com/leaders/2023/11/16/donald-trump-poses-the-biggest-danger-to-the-world-in-2024

Green, L. (2022a, September 16). The *Divider* review: Riveting narrative of Trump's plot against America. *Guardian.* Retrieved from https://www.theguardian.com/books/2022/sep/16/the-divider-review-donald-trump-peter-baker-susan-glasser.

Green, L. (2022b, December 11). 'That's Hitler, Bannon thought': 2022 in books about Trump and U.S. politics. *Guardian.* Retrieved from https://www.theguardian.com/books/2022/dec/11/trump-books-2022-politics-bestsellers-haberman-woodward.

Lee, B. X. (2017). *The Dangerous Case of Donald Trump: 27 Psychiatrists and Mental Health Experts Assess a President.* New York, NY: St. Martin's Press.

Lee, B. X. (2019). *The Dangerous Case of Donald Trump: 37 Psychiatrists and Mental*

Health Experts Assess a President. New York, NY: St. Martin's Press.

Lee, B. X. (2020). *Profile of a Nation: Trump's Mind, America's Soul.* New York, NY: World Mental Health Coalition.

Lee, B. X. (2024). *The Psychology of Trump Contagion: An Existential Danger to American Democracy and All Humankind.* New York, NY: World Mental Health Coalition.

Lindsey, R., and Dahlman, L. (2024, January 18). *Climate Change: Global Temperature.* Washington, DC: National Oceanic and Atmospheric Administration. https://www.climate.gov/news-features/understanding-climate/climate-change-global-temperature

PART 1
THANATOS
(DEATH DRIVE)

PRE-SENTENCING REPORT ON CONVICTED CRIMINAL DONALD J. TRUMP

JAMES GILLIGAN, M.D., JUDITH LEWIS HERMAN, M.D., ROBERT JAY LIFTON, M.D., JAMES R. MERIKANGAS, M.D., AND BANDY X. LEE, M.D., M.DIV.

(This is a reproduction of the original dangerousness risk assessment that was submitted to the Manhattan District Commissioner of Probation and Justice Juan Merchan on June 17, 2024, printed here for the purpose of public education.)

We are all psychiatrists with extensive experience in assessing the past and future dangerousness of criminal offenders and/or in working with the consequences of criminal violence. As co-authors of *The Dangerous Case of Donald Trump: 37 Psychiatrists and Mental Health Experts Assess a President* (2017 and 2019), we have already assessed the dangers that Donald Trump posed to this country and the world, as of the times in which we wrote the two editions of that book—all of which he has more than demonstrated in the years since. We donated all book revenues to the public good to remove conflicts of interest. We met with over fifty members of Congress "to serve society by advising and consulting with the executive, legislative, and judicial branches of the government" on medical matters, in accordance with our code of ethics. We now offer our recommendations for use at the time of sentencing, as a part of our professional societal responsibility and as a service to the public.

One of the main purposes of a pre-sentencing report or evaluation, as we under-

3

stand it, is to provide information that can help the court to determine the degree to which a person convicted of breaking a law or laws, especially if they are crimes that rise to the level of felonies, presents a risk of repeating the same or similar crimes—and even worse, of committing further, more serious crimes. In this context, mental health experts are routinely consulted for proper adjudication. We are frequently asked to evaluate dangerousness or violence risk and regularly testify in courts with the results of our findings. We employ standardized techniques and scientifically-validated scales to assess risk. We take into consideration direct violence, capability of instigating violence, and ability to harm the public's health.

Let us begin, then, with noticing how serious the crimes were that this particular convicted criminal, Donald Trump, committed. For crimes that may appear to be the same verbally, such as committing "fraud," may in fact range from being those that do relatively little harm (so-called "white lies" or "white collar" misdemeanors), to deliberately and systematically attempting to subvert and suspend the Constitution of the United States and the rule of law, and to replace our democracy with a dictatorship.

Indeed, the lies and deceptions that Mr. Trump committed, in violation of election laws, to influence the election by depriving the electorate of important information about his character, did not consist merely of concealing the purpose of checks that he signed. They were as serious as any crimes that have ever been committed in the history of our country— namely, an attempt to destroy our democracy and replace it with a dictatorship.

That latter formula describes the criminal behavior that Trump was convicted of and will be sentenced for. We are not speculating when we say that. We are merely quoting, verbatim, what he himself has said about himself, repeatedly and publicly: namely, that his goal is to suspend the Constitution, to become a dictator from "day one," and to use the Department of Justice to persecute his enemies, should he be re-elected as president. And of course, no dictator has ever relinquished power voluntarily on the second day he was in power; on the contrary, dictators, virtually by definition, hold onto as much power as they can command, for as long as they can command it. That is what it means to be a dictator, namely, to command the law, rather than to be commanded by the law.

The difference between democracy and autocracy (a dictatorship or tyranny) is the difference between political power based on the will of "We the people" (*demos*)— and political power that is based on the will of one person, or one self (*autos*). Donald Trump has made it clear that he will tell any lies and commit any deception that he feels will increase his chances of becoming a dictator, and that he will not respect and acknowledge the results of any presidential election that he does not win (which is what it means to be a dictator). He has combined this with threats of using his dictatorial power to incite or even order his subordinates to incarcerate or even execute his political opponents, no matter who he decides they are, and however numerous he believes them to be.

Thus, this convicted criminal has openly written his own pre-sentencing report, the conclusion of which is that he will do whatever he has the power to do, in the future, to continue his attempt to subvert and destroy the U.S. Constitution, the democratic structure of our government, and the rule of law. He has continued to express his total lack of remorse for the crimes of which he has been convicted, which is one of the best predictors of the likelihood that he will continue to repeat those crimes, and to do so on an even larger scale, as he gains even more power to do so.

That is why the only way to protect our democracy and the convicted criminal's attempt to subvert it—the crime of which he has just been convicted—is to restrain him by any means that the laws of sentencing permit, up to and including incarceration, for as long as those laws permit. Anything less than that would be insufficient to protect our nation, and indeed the entire world, from criminal behavior on a scale that we have never seen before in our history, committed by a man who is totally unrepentant and uninhibited about doing so.

Standardized, evidence-based violence risk assessment tools agree with our conclusions. These are behavioral and actuarial measures that do not require an in-person interview. The convicted criminal scored 8 (from a score range of -26 to +38) on the Violence Risk Appraisal Guide–Revised (VRAG-R) and 35 (prorated at 36, from a maximum score of 40) on the Psychopathy Checklist–Revised (PCL-R). These scores are consistent with a full diagnosis of psychopathy, which is highly predictive of violence, and indicate a significant need for specific deterrence, or at least containment (even without consideration of the need for general deterrence, which the VRAG-R does not measure).

Psychopathy makes his history of criminal behavior likely to repeat, or even be surpassed by more serious crimes. It is also relevant and important to note his demonstrated incapacity to feel guilty for his crimes against others, his complete lack of remorse, his contempt of court as shown by his inciting violence against judge, jury, and prosecutors, and his attempt to reverse the meaning of his criminal conviction by claiming that it merely proved that the legal system itself was illegitimate—or in other words, that it was the legal system itself that was criminal, not himself.

In assessing his character, for purposes of sentencing, it is relevant to notice that he has been adjudicated in a civil court to have committed sexual assault—in effect, rape—concerning which, as with the crimes which this report concerns, he has also shown no remorse, and has treated the legal system that resulted in his conviction with the same degree of contempt for the rule of law that he has shown here.

Of the two types of deterrence for felonies—specific and general—general deterrence is of great significance, given Donald Trump's rhetoric and his influence on his millions of followers, many of whom echo and act out his message with violent behavior and even insurrection. Mr. Trump may not himself be deterrable, by any degree of punishment—he may only be restrainable, by incarceration. However, we would hope that his sentence would be sufficiently severe to communicate, as a message to his followers, how real, serious, illegitimate, and unacceptable his criminality was, and thus achieve the goal of general deterrence.

RECOMMENDATIONS

While power in itself is morally neutral, in that it can be used for good or bad purposes, it can be extremely dangerous when it is possessed by people who exhibit traits of psychopathy—habitually repeated dishonest, antisocial, violent, and criminal behavior—of which the convicted criminal here has scored dangerously high. Grandiosity can develop into full-blown delusions of grandeur, and psychopathic traits can be amplified when the leader of an authoritarian cult of personality finds that he can break the law with impunity. When such a leader finally faces accountability, he is likely to become even more vengeful and dangerous. All these traits are exacerbated when they accompany rapid cognitive decline, as Donald Trump may be demonstrating openly and publicly. Mr. Trump's threats should therefore be taken seriously, and his potential to cause catastrophic harm must be fully considered, given his potentially unique position of power. We believe our recommendations would be fully supported, should the court choose to order a complete in-person medical and psychiatric evaluation, as the rules permit, in a designated hospital for up to thirty days. In determining an appropriate sentence for the former president, the Court has a unique opportunity to protect public safety and national security by restraining him, as far as possible and for as long as possible, from continuing to attempt to subvert the rule of law and our democratic form of government.

Prepared on the 17th of June, 2024, by:
J.G., J.L.H., R.J.L., J.R.M., B.X.L.

James Gilligan, M.D., is a Clinical Professor of Psychiatry and an Adjunct Professor of Law at New York University. He is the author of Violence: Our Deadly Epidemic and Its Causes, Preventing Violence, *and* Why Some Politicians Are More Dangerous than Others. *While on the faculty of Harvard Medical School (1966-2001), he helped to organize highly successful violence-reduction programs, such as "the Boston Miracle." He was Chair of President Clinton's National Campaign Against Youth Violence, and served in a similar capacity for Tony Blair, the Secretary-General of the United Nations, the World Health Organization, the World Court, and the World Economic Forum.*

Judith Lewis Herman, M.D., is Senior Lecturer in Psychiatry at Harvard Medical School. She is a renowned expert in the traumas of interpersonal violence and author of the now classic Trauma and Recovery. *She is a Distinguished Life Fellow of the American Psychiatric Association and the recipient of numerous awards, including the Lifetime Achievement Award from International Society for Traumatic Stress Studies. Her most recent book,* Truth and Repair: How Trauma Survivors Envision Justice, *was published in 2023.*

Robert Jay Lifton, M.D., is Lecturer in Psychiatry at Columbia University and Distinguished Professor Emeritus of John Jay College and the Graduate Center of the City University of New York. A leading psycho-historian, his renown comes from his studies of the doctors who aided Nazi war crimes and from his work with Hiroshima survivors. He was an outspoken critic of the American Psychological Association's aiding of government-sanctioned torture, as he is a vocal opponent of nuclear weapons. His research encompasses the psychological causes and effects of war and political violence and the theory of thought reform.

James R. Merikangas, M.D., is a neuropsychiatrist, Cofounder of the American Neuropsychiatric Association, and former President of the American Academy of Clinical Psychiatrists. He graduated from Johns Hopkins University School of Medicine and trained in neurology and psy-

chiatry at Yale. Dr. Merikangas established the EEG laboratory at the Western Psychiatric Clinic of the University of Pittsburgh, where he also established the neurodiagnostic clinic and directed the psychiatric emergency room. Currently he is Clinical Professor of Psychiatry and Behavioral Science at George Washington University School of Medicine and Health Sciences and a Research Consultant at the National Institute of Mental Health.

Bandy X. Lee, M.D., M.Div., is a forensic and social psychiatrist and an internationally-recognized violence expert. She taught at Yale School of Medicine and Yale Law School (2003-2020) before joining the Harvard Program in Psychiatry and the Law. She authored the textbook, Violence: An Interdisciplinary Approach to Causes, Consequences, and Cures, *used in universities worldwide. She advised numerous state and national governments and international bodies on public health approaches to violence prevention, including the World Health Organization's landmark* World Report on Violence and Health. *She is President of the World Mental Health Coalition and Cofounder of the Violence Prevention Institute.*

THE IMPORTANT ISSUE IS VIOLENCE AND DANGEROUSNESS

James Gilligan, M.D.

It is cause for alarm, not satisfaction, that the warnings my colleagues and I made in 2016 as to the dangerousness of Donald Trump, even before he was elected, have been proven since then (by him) to have been so accurate, indeed prophetic—for he has proven that our predictions of his incitements to future violence and the overthrow of our democracy were, if anything, understated. The deadly, armed invasion of the U.S. Capitol Building on Jan. 6, 2021, by American insurrectionists (Trump's followers), and the forced evacuation of both Houses of Congress, was of course the most unprecedented attempt in American history to overthrow the most basic elements of our democratic system of government, and to replace them with those that underlie dictatorship—namely, force, violence, and coercion. Even the slave states of the South at the time of our Civil War, were only attempting to remain racial dictatorships in their own states, not to overthrow the democratic governments of the entire country, including those of the Northern states.

This is why I think the most important and relevant fact for us to recognize about Trump is his dangerousness, by which I mean his ability and willingness to incite political violence, and thus to replace democracy with dictatorship. For democracy is based on persuasion—of voters, legislators, judges, and juries—by means of evidence and rational analysis of evidence, by means of words, debate, and discussion; whereas, dictatorship is based on physical violence, force, and coercion—as exemplified by the attack on both Houses of Congress on January 6.

While I will discuss many of the ways in which Trump's public verbal behavior exemplifies symptoms of various different varieties of the mental disorders defined in the current Diagnostic and Statistical Manual of the American Psychiatric Association, I want to emphasize that this is not my main point. Most of those who are mentally ill never commit a serious act of violence in their lifetimes, and most of those who commit acts of lethal violence, such as homicides, are not mentally ill as that concept is defined both by the criminal law and by forensic psychiatry. (Only about one per cent of those who commit homicides are judged to be "not guilty by reason of insanity." All the others are presumed either to be mentally healthy, or at least not to have committed their homicides as a consequence of mental illness.)

But those who commit acts of violence, for whatever reason, are, by definition, dangerous; my main point here is that even if Trump meets the clinical criteria for a diagnosis of one or more forms of mental disorders, the most important and relevant question is not, "Is he mentally ill or not, and if so, with what diagnosis?"; but rather, "How dangerous is he—regardless of diagnosis?"

Since his election to the presidency in 2016, and his loss in 2020, he has bragged that he would become a "dictator" on the first day of his renewed presidency (in 2025); that he might find it "necessary" to suspend the Constitution of the United States; and that he would prosecute those who dared to disagree with him, such as General Mark Milley and an indefinite but expandable catalogue of others, whom he accuses of treason (a crime punishable by death). He has threatened to turn the U.S. military into his personal police force, subjecting American citizens to their violence, and to declare a state of emergency in order to do so. And, as I've said, his incitement of the deadly, armed invasion (or attempted, but failed, *coup d'etat*) at the Capitol on January 6, 2021, was an attempt to replace democracy (regime change by means of elections) with dictatorship (the *prevention* of regime change, by means of *violence*).

Indeed, his appetite for violence is so insatiable, his sense of personal entitlement is so unlimited, and his hypocrisy is so gargantuan, that this faux-billionaire, who has a history of property crimes on the scale of millions of dollars, has advocated that even the most trivial of property crimes—shoplifting—should be punishable by the death penalty!

It should be remembered that the most dangerous mass-murderous dictators in history—Hitler, Mussolini, Stalin, Mao, etc.—may have killed no one—or at most a few people—themselves. They have gone down in history as the architects of the deadliest political violence in human history not because they themselves killed anyone, but because they incited their followers to commit millions of murders for them. By the same token, Trump himself may never have killed a single individual. But he has certainly incited his followers to do this for him, and not only on January 6.

It is even more important to notice that in this era of thermonuclear weapons, Trump has incomparably more destructive power than even the most homicidal of past dictators. Even Hitler and Stalin were only capable of genocide. The President of the United States, as Commander-in-Chief of the military, has the power to commit human-icide.

I realize most people believe that even if he ordered the use of thermonuclear weapons (as he has in fact, on more than one occasion, threatened to do), military leaders would be rational and humane enough to refuse to follow his orders. But that assumes he did not mean it when he said that he would replace such leaders with those who would do whatever he wanted.

As for Trump's mental status, the fact that President Biden has decided not to run for re-election, after revealing in his debate with Trump that he sometimes had trouble finishing sentences (and some other "soft" signs of aging), has had the effect of eliminat-ing the double standard that had existed up to then: namely, the fact that the media was paying attention to the signs of Biden's loss of mental acuity, but ignoring the fact that Trump (only four years younger) has even more glaring difficulties fashioning coherent sentences, arguments, and answers to questions. Clearly, Trump has many more symp-toms of dementia than Biden ever had.

Whether he is demented or not, there is another, perhaps even more important question about Trump's mental status. And that is, how are we to understand his unre-lenting repetition of untruths? The *Washington Post*, among other observers of his verbal behavior, has documented tens of thousands of public statements by Trump that are obvi-ous and well-documented distortions, or outright denials, of well-proven factual realities.

It seems to me that there are only two reasonable interpretations of this behavior on his part. As a psychiatrist, I have been trained to recognize that the "denial" of real-ity (i.e., being "out of touch with" reality), is one of the most damaging and dangerous cognitive distortions, or defense mechanisms, that people who suffer from one form or another of psychopathology exhibit. Therefore, the question is: does Trump believe in the denials of obvious, everyday reality that he expresses verbally (in which case they are called delusions of persecution, of grandeur, etc. –which are symptoms of psychotic illnesses such as paranoia, schizophrenia, or mania) –or does he know they are false but utters them anyway, in which case he is chronically, constantly, habitually lying—which is a symptom of another form of psychopathology, called psychopathy, sociopathy, or

11

antisocial character disorder: persistent lying, as a means of manipulating, deceiving, and gaining power over other people, in order to exploit or abuse them.

But in either case, regardless of whether Trump's untruthful statements are delusions or lies, they indicate how dangerous he would be as President of the United States.

But that raises another question: how could millions of voters, who are neither mentally ill, dishonest, or ignorant themselves, believe Trump's untruthful assertion that he in fact won the 2020 presidential election (despite the fact that 30 different courts, throughout the country, were unanimous in finding no evidence of that being true)? How could they chant, "Stop the steal!", when the presidency has repeatedly and unanimously been proven in 30 different courts of law *not* to have been stolen from Trump?

To answer that question, I think it will be useful to recall the psychiatric syndrome described by 19th century French psychiatrists, which they called "*Folie a deux*" ("madness of two")—a delusional belief shared by two people. What that term was used to describe and identify was a phenomenon they occasionally observed clinically (and which I have seen in my own clinical practice), in which one powerful and influential member of a family—say, a parent or spouse—develops a psychotic delusion, such as a delusion of persecution, ("The police, or our neighbors, are spying on us," or, "Our thoughts are being controlled by outside forces"); and a less powerful and more dependent, influenceable, but not independently psychotic family member believes that idea is a truthful description of reality. Thus, it becomes a kind of shared delusion of persecution.

But—and this is the important point—they discovered that when the dependent person is separated from the more powerful psychotic family member, they stop believing in the delusion, and regain their normal, healthy capacity for "reality testing."

I believe something comparable to that is going on in Trump's capacity to induce millions of normal, sane, honest, and knowledgeable people—i.e., Trump voters—to share his delusion (or believe his lie) that he won the 2020 election. We could call this not a "Folie a deux," but a "Folie aux millions."

The clearest historical analogy to this phenomenon, I would suggest, is the shared, collective delusion of persecution on which Nazism was based -- i.e., that the Jews were persecuting and endangering the Germans, and that the Germans needed to exterminate the Jews in order to defend themselves.

Once Hitler was removed from the scene, the Germans regained their capacity for reality-testing, dropped that collective, shared delusion of persecution (and the associated delusion of grandeur, namely, that Germans were the "master race"), and have become one of the most stable and rational democracies in the world. (Though they, like the U.S., have also suffered from the resurgence of political movements that currently threaten— though unsuccessfully so far -- to bring about a regression to a slightly updated version of that same old collective psychosis—typically, as in this country, in regions and among sub-groups that are suffering from declining levels of relative affluence and social status, and hence from painful feelings of inferiority, or shame).

Trump's version of this ethnocentrism and xenophobia includes his repeated allegations that immigrants (from Latin America, Muslim countries, etc.) are more likely to commit violent crimes than those born in this country, and that violent crime increases when Democrats are in power, and decreases when Republicans are.

In fact, both of those allegations are not merely untrue—that is, they are not exaggerations of minor but true differences—they are the exact, diametrical *opposite* of the truth; immigrants commit *lower* rates of criminal violence than native-born Americans do. And lethal violence rates (homicide and suicide) have cumulatively, collectively, and significantly *increased*, since 1900 (i.e., during the past 120 years) during Republican presidential administrations, and *decreased* during Democratic ones (Gilligan, 2011; Lee, Wexler and Gilligan, 2014). So, he is not *exaggerating* the truth, he is *reversing* it.

To put it in other terms, he is *projecting*—onto immigrants and Democrats— characteristics that are true of him and his associates, and clearly *untrue* of those he is accusing of possessing these characteristics. (Projection—accusing others of doing what you yourself are doing— is a mechanism of defense that is central both to paranoia and to psychopathic lying.)

My hope is that if and when Trump is defeated in the 2024 election, he will have been removed from the political sphere enough for those who had believed in his untruths (e.g., that Democrats had stolen his elections from him) to regain their normal capacity for reality-testing, and drop those false, indeed grossly unrealistic and repeatedly, consistently refuted beliefs, just as the non-psychotic partners who had shared a *Folie a deux* regained their innate capacity for normal reality-testing once they were separated from their psychotic, but influential, family member. On the other hand, if Trump does win the election, I can only fear for the future, not only of this country, but of the rest of the world as well.

James Gilligan, M.D., is a Clinical Professor of Psychiatry and an Adjunct Professor of Law at New York University. He is the author of Violence: Our Deadly Epidemic and Its Causes, Preventing Violence, *and* Why Some Politicians Are More Dangerous than Others. *While on the faculty of Harvard Medical School (1966-2001), he helped to organize highly successful violence-reduction programs, such as "the Boston Miracle." He was Chair of President Clinton's National Campaign Against Youth Violence, and served in a similar capacity for Tony Blair, the Secretary-General of the United Nations, the World Health Organization, the World Court, and the World Economic Forum.*

References

Gilligan, J. (2011). *Why Some Politicians Are More Dangerous than Others*. Cambridge, U.K.: Polity Press.

Lee, B. X., Wexler, B. E., and Gilligan, J. (2014). Political correlates of violent death rates in the u.s., 1900-2010: Longitudinal and cross-sectional analyses," *Aggression and Violent Behavior*, 19:721-728.

DONALD TRUMP, LIKE HITLER, IS A PSYCHOPATH

Lance Dodes, M.D.

In the first edition of this book, I wrote a chapter titled "Sociopathy" to describe the many reasons Donald Trump fits the definition of a sociopath, a term that describes the characteristics of Antisocial Personality Disorder. Now, with the evidence of more years of his criminality, his incredible and continuous lying, his absence of empathy (incapacity for concern for anyone but himself), and, currently, his willingness to sacrifice democracy and the freedom of the people for his own benefit, there are enough data to confirm that Trump exhibits the most severe traits associated with Antisocial Personality Disorder—that he is a psychopath. This is by far the most dangerous of all mental disorders, since it is the only psychological condition in which behaving in a morally reprehensible way is an essential part of its nature.

Psychopaths intentionally create harm to others without guilt or remorse, for personal gain or self-gratification. That gratification often includes the sadistic pleasure of wreaking revenge against imagined enemies. Psychopaths cannot be reasoned out of their beliefs or their behavior, because they are unable to comprehend that others have value, or the concept of questioning themselves. The fact that Donald Trump has this most dangerous form of Antisocial Personality Disorder has two long-term consequences: It means that he is never going to stop intentionally harming others for his personal benefit, and it means that he will become worse over time.

Trump as a tyrant

With his use of the Big Lie technique, attacks on minorities and immigrants, and claims that only he can save America, Trump has shown that he is following the very same plan as Hitler and other truly evil dictators in human history.

One of the characteristics of these tyrants is something that distinguishes psychopaths from sociopaths. Beyond lawbreaking, lying, cheating, and the absence of conscience, psychopaths are known for their long-term planning to intentionally harm others. Trump's conviction on multiple counts of fraud, his inciting violence toward political opponents and officers of the courts, and his plan to violently overthrow the government of the United States on January 6, 2021, show the planned, intentional, criminal nature of his thinking. Like the abhorrent tyrants of the past, he is willing for other people to be denied their rights in order for him to have power, and he is eager to vengefully abuse people when it suits his purposes.

The following three statements were made not by Donald Trump but by Adolf Hitler, yet they uncannily describe Trump's pathological behavior, thinking, and attitude toward others:

- "Strength lies not in defense but in attack."
- "I cannot be mistaken—what I say and do is historical."
- "The masses are more likely to believe a big lie than a little one."

As Trump has shown numerous times when he is questioned, rather than having a rational response, he insults and mocks those who dare to challenge him. He has never acknowledged mistakes; indeed, he has repeatedly described himself as godlike. He has told enormous lies over and over, such as that he won the last election, with the intention that by repetition, he will fool the people into believing him.

Trump's lack of humanity

Trump's absence of concern for others, and longstanding efforts to control and sadistically attack others, set him apart from normal human beings. What we often admire about ourselves as a species is our ability to care for and about one another, come to the aid of our fellow human, and join in shared efforts to help all of us. As a consequence, society normally does not tolerate individuals like Donald Trump who incite violence and abuse others for their self-interest. We would have expected society to protect itself from him. His recent conviction on more than 30 counts of fraud is an example of an attempt to do just that. But the power of conscience-free manipulation, coupled with the Big Lie technique, has, many times in human history, proven to overcome people's normal self-preservation when practiced by a convincing psychopath. This happened to the people of Germany in the 1930's when they surrendered a vibrant democracy to the lies and false promises of their psychopath. Now, the people of America are at risk of repeating this tragedy.

Conclusion

With his public admission that he intends to be a dictator, saying there will be no more need to vote once he seizes power, the danger from Donald Trump has become lethal for democracy. Trump's exhibiting the most severe characteristics of Antisocial Personality Disorder—his being a psychopath—is why he threatens, hurts, debases, and attempts to control others for his own benefit, and why he will never change but, instead, will become worse the more power he can seize.

Trump is America's Hitler because Trump and Hitler are not only both psychopaths, but Trump has intentionally followed Hitler's plan of endless repetition of Big Lies such as that the 2020 election was "stolen" from him. He has repeatedly threatened and criminally acted his way to power through violence and attempts to corrupt the nation's legal and electoral systems. Like other historic scourges of humanity, Trump has shown that he falls far beneath the hallmark of mutual caring that makes us human.

Democracy requires respect and protection for multiple points of view, concepts that are impossible for psychopaths. If we are to survive as a free country, we all need to understand the depth of psychological illness of Donald Trump, and the absence of morality that arises from his most severe mental illness.

Lance Dodes, M.D., is a Training and Supervising Analyst Emeritus at the Boston Psychoanalytic Society and Institute, and retired Assistant Clinical Professor of Psychiatry at Harvard Medical School. He is the author of many academic articles and book chapters describing a new understanding of the nature and treatment of addiction, and three books: The Heart of Addiction; Breaking Addiction; *and* The Sober Truth. *He has been honored by the Division on Addictions at Harvard Medical School for "Distinguished Contribution" to the study and treatment of addictive behavior, and has been elected a Distinguished Fellow of the American Academy of Addiction Psychiatry.*

TRUMP IS A PSYCHOPATH
The Hare Psychopathy Checklist

VINCE GREENWOOD, PH.D., AND SETH D. NORRHOLM, PH.D.

Shortly after Trump's election in 2016, many mental health professionals, including several authors of this volume, spoke out about the new president's unfitness for office. They linked Trump's behaviors with distinct psychological patterns that result in harm to others. The World Mental Health Coalition[1], under the supervision of Bandy Lee, published *The Dangerous Case of Donald Trump*[2], an edited volume of appraisals of Trump's dangerous psychopathology. The public seemed to have an appetite for insight into Trump's psyche, as evidenced by the appearance of the book on the *New York Times* bestseller list.

Government officials, pundits and television media personalities have routinely described the 45th President as "nuts[3]," "out of his mind[4]," or "crazy[5]." In addition, there has been considerable debate regarding psychiatric diagnoses, the Goldwater Rule[6], and the so-called "Duty to Warn,[7]" which has been placed on mental health professionals whose patients or clients reveal malicious, harmful, violent, or deadly intentions. Perhaps it would be appropriate to add a "Duty to Inform" principle that holds that mental health experts have a duty to inform the public about meaningful, objectively clear, and dangerous health issues regarding those running for higher office.

Were these efforts to warn impactful? Many voters considered the election an existential moment for the country, and warnings from professionals validated that concern. It certainly seemed that the input from the mental health community was one of the factors contributing to Trump's defeat.

And yet…for many of us in the mental health community, it seemed like our findings should have had a greater impact. After all, many of us had spelled out psychological disturbances that demonstrated Trump was unfit for office, clinically dangerous, and really was an existential threat. In fact, Dr. Norrholm, in collaboration with a colleague, published an opinion piece in the New York Daily News that explicitly stated, 'The President is a Psychopath[8].' Dr. Greenwood has been educating the public about psychopathy through his organization, Duty to Inform (DutytoInform.org), since 2020. Given those findings, how could the election have even been close?

Since election night in 2020, we have witnessed the attack on the Capitol, the shredding of democratic norms (most notably the peaceful transfer of power), a deep polarization that has become a cold civil war, and an assault on the concept of truth that Lee depicts in her recent book, *The Psychology of Trump Contagion*[9]. Several factors contribute to our current political crisis, but the impact of Trump's psychiatric condition is the crucial ingredient. His psychopathology reverberates through our body politic.

That psychopathology takes a number of forms, but perhaps the most consequential is his personality disorder. Donald Trump suffers from a precisely delineated psychiatric condition called Psychopathic Personality Disorder[10]. He is at the mercy of a set of destructive personality traits that make up that condition. That is quite sad for him, but also quite dangerous for the rest of us. Indeed, as mental health professionals, we have an ethical duty to inform you that, even with all he has done and all he has threatened to do, because of his condition, we are on solid scientific grounds to warn you that we are underestimating the danger he poses.

Such a serious assertion requires a detailed and evidence-based explanation.

Let's start with a bit of history[11] on this dangerous disorder. This condition has been with us from antiquity through medieval times to the present. Descriptions from Greek and Roman mythology, the Bible, and classical literature are remarkably consistent in revealing the presence of a small group among us that are intellectually coherent but lack the capacity for moral reasoning. Such individuals do not seem to experience emotional suffering— there is no psychosis, no anxiety, no depression— and seem impervious to punishment. They display a constellation of personality traits frequently associated with immorality and criminality, but also, in some cases, socioeconomic success, even if that success is gained through dishonest means. No culture or station in life is immune from this condition. It is described across all of written history, and we find it among the wealthy and the impoverished.

Our understanding of such individuals took a quantum leap in the 20th century due primarily to the work of two men. Hervey Cleckley, an American psychiatrist from

Georgia, devoted his career to studying this condition and published his insights in a book titled *The Mask of Sanity*[12] in 1941. Considered one of the great works in the field of psychopathology, it depicted the psychopath as an individual, while appearing to be a perfectly average person, indeed often a charming person, who nevertheless displays a particular set of traits which inevitably lead to menacing behavioral patterns that are harmful to others. The harm manifests itself at times in criminal acts, but always in exploitive behavior, marked by arrogance, cunning and deceit.

In the 1970s, Robert Hare, a Canadian psychologist, and his research team developed a checklist to diagnose the condition. This measurement tool is called the **Hare Psychopathy Checklist**[13]. The Checklist triggered an explosion of studies. Google Scholar now cites some 83,000 studies associated with the Checklist, enabling us to develop a detailed and scientific understanding of the condition. That research has validated the descriptions from classical literature; there is a distinct condition that afflicts a small number of us that is stable across history, culture, and socioeconomic status. Psychopathic Personality Disorder is not just a term of disapprobation for (mostly) men behaving very badly, but a diagnosis that reflects a real world, clearly defined pathogen with predictable consequences. Because the Hare Psychopathy Checklist_enabled us to objectively measure the condition, we can now say that clinical psychopathy is one of the most thoroughly validated and best-understood conditions in the field of psychopathology.

We need to discuss the Psychopathy Checklist briefly to understand why we can speak with depth and specificity about Donald Trump's dangerousness.
The Psychopathy Checklist has 20 items. These items reflect the very problematic but stable and long-standing traits and behavior patterns that Hervey Cleckley and some other leading experts in the field had identified. For each item, the diagnostician is asked to give a rating on the pervasiveness of the trait. The guidelines to diagnose psychopathy are straightforward, but the demands on the diagnostician are rigorous.

First, you are required to collect voluminous data, basically detailed life history information. The diagnostic process for this condition demands:

(1) Information from the patient's childhood, adolescence, and young adulthood, since the condition of psychopathy expresses itself early in life;
(2) Life history information in which the trait is expressed in observable. behavior (e.g., evidence of lying is preferable to the accusation of his lying);
(3) Information that reflects the patient's typical functioning and lifelong patterns,

rather than descriptions of more flamboyant, occasional behavior; and

(4) Well-resourced information with some type of external validation.

Second, you are required to undergo specialized training to administer the Checklist. The training involves learning extensive definitions and behavioral examples of checklist items; how to collect and evaluate the quality-of-life history information from different sources; securing feedback on videotaped case studies to increase precision on the administration of the checklists; and other skills to ensure a reliable and valid diagnosis.

For each item, you get a score of 0 (no meaningful expression of the trait in the person's life), 1 (moderate expression of the trait), or 2 (strong expression of the trait— it is persistent and pervasive in the person's life). With 20 items, a perfect score on the psychopathy end of the spectrum would be 40 (a very rare occurrence), and a perfect score on the non-psychopathy side would be 0 (also rare).

For the evaluation of Donald Trump, we first need to ask and answer the question: Can you diagnose someone for clinical psychopathy at a distance? A strong "yes" is answered if you have sufficient life history data. Fortunately, with Trump, we are awash with information. He is arguably the most well-chronicled candidate in history. A partial list of informational sources would include 13 autobiographical efforts as well as his social media posts, 71 biographies, many of which are richly sourced, and hundreds of interviews from print, radio, and television. A clinical interview is not necessary to diagnose the former president for this condition. Indeed, there is research to indicate that the interview can detract from the assessment of a psychopath because of their facility for lying.[14]

Before we present the findings on Trump, please note the average score for someone in the general population is 5[15]. The average score for individuals in a maximum-security prison setting is 22. I mention that because the typical cutoff to get a formal diagnosis of psychopathy is 30. It's a high bar that even most serious criminals don't meet.

With these anchor points in mind here are the ratings for Trump on the Psychopathy Checklist:

Hare Psychopathy Checklist-Revised (PCL-R)
1. Glibness/superficial charm— 2

2 Egocentricity/grandiose sense of self-worth— 2

3. Proneness to boredom/need for stimulation— 2

4. Pathological lying and deception/gaslighting— 2

5. Conning/lack of sincerity— 2

6. Lack of remorse or guilt— 2

7. Shallow affect— 2

8. Callous/lack of empathy— 2

9. Parasitic lifestyle— 1

10. Poor behavioral controls— 2

11. Promiscuous sexual behavior— 2

12. Early behavior problems— 2

13. Lack of realistic long-term goals— 1

14. Impulsivity— 2

15. Irresponsibility— 2

16. Failure to accept responsibility for own actions— 2

17. Many short-term marital relationships— 1

18. Juvenile delinquency— 1

19. Revocation of parole— 0

20. Criminal versatility— 2

Total = 34

Trump receives a score of 34. Remarkably, another scoring by a panel of five psychiatrists (Drs. Robert Jay Lifton, Judith Herman, James Gilligan, James Merikan-gas, and Bandy Lee), as part of a pre-sentencing report to the Manhattan Criminal Court following Donald Trump's felony conviction, yielded a remarkably close score of 35, which they prorated to 36, given the absence of prior convictions. This demonstrates the reliability and consistency of the scale, as proven across numerous studies.

The diagnostic process to assess clinical psychopathy demands thoroughness and objectivity. This rating reflects a fair-minded effort to call balls and strikes. Donald Trump passes the threshold for a formal diagnosis of clinical psychopathy.

What does this diagnosis tell us? What have we learned about the condition? We have learned that the condition is more due to nature (what one inherits) than nurture (how the environment impacts us), and that what is largely inherited appears to be a different brain. Brain imaging technology[16] has enabled us to pinpoint some of the distinctive features in the brains of psychopaths that help explain their hard-wired traits.

Most critically (and most relevant to the appraisal of Trump), we have achieved insight into the essence of the disorder, what psychologists call the deep structure of the condition.

How do you go about zeroing in on the essence of a psychiatric condition? The challenge with a large and expanding data set, like that which exists for clinical psychopathy, is to find a way to distill it. Investigators turned to factor analysis, a robust data reduction technique that enables us to explore and identify primary, underlying factors in a large data set. It is a tool often used in personality research to reduce findings of many specific traits, behavioral observations, and other meaningful data points into more basic underlying factors or clusters of traits.

What has come out of the empirical wash with these solidly-built statistical techniques is the clarity that the psychopath is ruled by three distinct clusters of traits (known as the "three factor model[17]" of clinical psychopathy). The three core, governing traits of the psychopath are:

(1) **Impulsivity**— characterized by the inability to inhibit impulses or grapple with any issue that doesn't serve the psychopath's immediate, egocentric needs.

(2) **Drive to dominate**— characterized by a one-dimensional focus on "winning" in all relationships, fueled by an arrogant, manipulative, and deceitful mode of behavior.

(3) **Remorselessness**— characterized by an utter lack of conscience, linked to an inability to experience states of guilt, shame, and fear that might curb immoral behavior.

All of the behavior and all of the choices of the psychopath flow from these three governing traits; thus:

Because of his **impulsivity**, Trump can't help but:
Act quickly without considering the consequences;
Take huge risks since he craves sensation-seeking;
Continue to display no aptitude for governance; and
Fail to plan or persevere with any substantive task

Because of his **drive to dominate**, Trump can't help but:

Lie with impunity to get others to bend to his will;

Demand fealty from others;

Engage in frantic efforts to avoid loss of status;

Foment divisiveness and polarization, and

Privilege power and dominance over the welfare of others;

Because of his **remorselessness**, Trump can't help but:

Blithely ignore democratic norms, the tragedy of lost lives, or appeals from any-one to rein in his reckless and derelict behavior;

Set any limits on his behavior since he is undaunted by the fear of punishment;

Deflect all responsibility for any damage he may inflict;

Have no feeling of discomfort at the suffering of others, and

Be lax in his response to legitimate threats because of his inability to process emotions related to danger.

In conclusion, like any diagnosed psychopath/malignant narcissist, Donald Trump has had to suffer a life devoid of love, depth, conscience, or any hope of self-discipline. It is a life incapable of developing a caring obligation toward others, incapable of remorse for callous or immoral behavior, and incapable of pursuing anything beyond his immediate self-interest.

It should be noted that Trump's psychopathy currently resides in a sociopolitical climate that is permissive of his actions and behaviors; phenomena once thought to be too antisocial, too sociopathic, or too psychopathic for a candidate or politician to thrive in *society* let alone an election campaign or term of office. Previously, such actors often experienced a need to disguise or hide sociopathic proclivities, but currently there is neither shame nor hesitation in openly acting in the service of sociopathy. The thing about malignant narcissists, sociopaths, psychopaths, and/or antisocial personalities is that if there are no legal, social, or occupational consequences, then their feeling of impunity (which *should* be a cognitive distortion) is validated as "having been correct all along"—a reason for prideful display and *continuation* of harmful behaviors.

Taken together, Trump's is a life destined to inflict harm and suffering on others. With the empirical support of thousands of studies on his condition, we have to warn that

Donald Trump, because of his hard-wired and immutable traits, is *more dangerous than even his harshest critics exclaim.*

Vince Greenwood, Ph.D., is the Founder and Executive Director of the Washington Center for Cognitive Therapy, a mental health practice that specializes in the treatment of anxiety and mood disorders. He has served as a consultant at the National Institute of Mental Health (NIMH) and Johns Hopkins University Hospital. He created Duty to Inform (Dutyto-Inform.org) in 2020, a website devoted to the intersection of psychology and politics.

Seth D. Norrholm, Ph.D., is the Director of the Neuroscience Center for Anxiety, Stress, and Trauma in Detroit, Michigan. Dr. Norrholm is a translational neuroscientist and psychologist with 24 years of research and clinical experience in the neurobiological mechanisms underlying fear-, anxiety-, trauma-, and stressor-related disorders. Specializing in psychological trauma, Dr. Norrholm studies long-term neuropsychobiological consequences of adverse life experiences including domestic abuse, and violent crime including analyzing contributing factors like nature, nurture, personality, and sociopolitical climate. He has authored over 140 peer-reviewed journal articles and book chapters, and is recognized as a world leader in posttraumatic stress disorder (PTSD).

References

1. World Mental Health Coalition. (2017). https://worldmhc.org/
2. *The Dangerous Case of Donald Trump: 27 Psychiatrists and Mental Health Experts Assess a President.* New York: St. Martin's Press, (2017).
3. https://www.cbsnews.com/news/trump-impeachment-nuts-kinzinger/ Segers, G. (2021). "GOP Congressman Adam Kinzinger says Trump is "nuts" after impeachment vote."
4. Reich, R. (2024). "Trump is out of his mind—and his speech in Ohio shows it." RawStory.com. https://www.rawstory.com/trumps-speech-in-ohio/

5. Olbermann, K. *Trump is F*cking Crazy*. New York, NY: Penguin Random House LLC, (2017).

6. McLoughlin, A. "The Goldwater Rule: a bastion of a bygone era?" *History of Psychiatry 2022*; 33(1):87-94.

7. California TvRoUo. 17 Cal.3d 425. In: California SCo, ed.1976.

8. Blotcky, A, Norrholm, SD. (2020). "Say it plainly: the president is a psychopath." The New York Daily News.

9. Lee, Bandy X. *The Psychology of Trump Contagion: An Existential Threat to American Democracy and All Humankind*. New York: World Mental Health Coalition, Inc. (2024).

10. Greenwood, Vincent. *A DUTY TO DIFFERENTIALLY DIAGNOSE: The Substance Behind the Assertion the President Has a Serious Psychiatric Condition.* https://drvincentgreenwood-89455.medium.com/a-duty-to-differentially-diagnose-the-validity-underpinning-the-diagnosis-of-the-president-cda2445963bf. 2020.

11. Kiehl, Kent and Hoffman, Morris. "The Criminal Psychopath: History, Neuroscience, Treatment, and Economics*." Journal of the National Library of Medicine, Summer*; 51: 355-397, 2011.

12. Cleckley, Hervey. *Mask of Sanity.* United States: Mobley Press, 1982.

13. Hare, Robert D. *Psychopathy Checklist—Revised.* APA PsycTests. https://doi.org/10.1037/t01167-000. 1991.

14. Porter, S., ten Brinke, L., and Wilson, K. "Crime profiles and conditional release performance of psychopathic and non-psychopathic sexual offenders*". Legal and Criminological Psychology*, 14(1), 109–118. (2009).

15. Kiehl, Kent and Hoffman, Morris. "The Criminal Psychopath: History, Neuroscience, Treatment, and Economics." *Journal of the National Library of Medicine, Summer*; 51: 355-397, 2011.

16. Kiehl, Kent A. *Psychopath Whisperer. The Science of Those Without Conscience.* The Crown Publishing Group, 2015.

17. Croom, Simon and Svetina, Marko. "Psychometric properties of the psychopathic personality inventory: Application to high-functioning business population*." Current Psychology*, 42(2), 2021.

IS TRUMP IN THE THROES OF EARLY DEMENTIA?

VINCE GREENWOOD, PH.D.

What would it mean if Donald Trump were suffering from a deteriorating neurological syndrome rather than just the typical alterations of aging? The mild decline in memory, attention, and verbal fluency associated with normal aging often emerges as one reaches their late 70s or early 80s. Such a decline would not necessarily be disqualifying, even regarding the demanding responsibilities of the presidency. However, a diagnosis of a deteriorating neurological disorder would have profound implications for his fitness for office. If the ex-president crossed that fateful diagnostic threshold, the public would have a right to be informed and a reason to be alarmed.

Although many observers have commented on Donald Trump's verbal and cognitive struggles over the past couple of years, conventional wisdom has concluded it is simply not possible to make a valid diagnosis of neurological decline with Trump. Good faith investigative reporters and health care professionals cite two reasons: The lack of medical information released by Trump and his doctors, and the inherent limitations of "diagnosing at a distance," which is the only resort available since Trump has refused a comprehensive neuropsychological examination.

We need to address these reasonable objections. A recent New York Times article, "What Are We Told About the Health of Biden and Trump? They Decide", captures this frustration.[1] Trump and his medical team have gone out of their way *not* to provide detailed information. His most recent report (November 2023) is a three-paragraph statement where his physician described his health as "excellent."[2] Earlier health reports have been criticized as "fawning and vague,"[3] marked by the use of superlatives ("the healthiest individual ever elected to the presidency"), and lack of details.[4]

And full of disinformation. Here, we need to mention Trump's assertions about a "cognitive test" he took in 2018, the Montreal Cognitive Assessment Test (MoCA). The MoCa, a one-page, 30-point test administered in 10 minutes, is an *initial* screening device that can detect signs of full-scale dementia. It's not helpful in identifying signs of early dementia, which requires more rigorous and lengthy testing. Trump reported a perfect score of 30, claiming doctors told him, "Rarely can anybody do what you just did," and that the test contains "very hard" questions.[5] The average score on the test is 27 (and even that average is from a sample of people suspected of cognitive impairment). A score of 30 is considered normal, not exceptional. Examples of questions from the supposedly tricky part of the test include repeating a sentence out loud; naming as many words as you can starting with the letter F; trying to identify the similarity between different objects such as trains and bicycles (modes of transportation); and saying what the current date is. Dr. Jonathan Reiner, professor of Medicine at George Washington Hospital, wryly observed, "If you think a dementia screening test is very difficult, you may have early dementia."[6]

We are not able to make a serious appraisal of whether Trump does or does not display brain illness based on his released medical records, since they lack any specificity and have been politicized.

Since Trump has refused to collaborate in a comprehensive neuropsychological exam, which would yield a wealth of relevant data, we must "diagnose at a distance" to try to determine the possibility of meaningful cognitive decline. A recent Washington Post article, "What Science Tells Us about Biden, Trump and Evaluating an Aging Brain," outlines the limitations.[7] Experts interviewed for that story assert that an informed opinion on the ex-president's cognitive health is only possible with the robust data generated from an in-depth exam. They note, correctly, that video mashups of verbal gaffes lack scientific rigor and can be misleading. Such mashups on social media can be guilty of cherry-picking bad moments and equating signs of normal aging with severe cognitive decline.

Are we forced to throw up our hands at the possibility of providing a more scientific and objective opinion about whether Trump suffers from a neurocognitive disorder?

The answer is no. *There is a legitimate path to arrive at an informed, scientifically-based opinion on Trump's brain health. That path involves subjecting all the relevant information to the guidelines enumerated in the chapter on Neurocognitive Disorders in the latest version of the Diagnostic and Statistical Manual of Mental Disorders. When we carry out those diagnostic steps, we find that Trump very likely has a Neurocognitive*

Disorder that is already beginning to have its way with his cognitive functioning and is destined to deteriorate, perhaps significantly, over the next few years.

Such a serious assertion demands a serious explanation. Let's start with the scientific standing of the diagnostic bible of the mental health profession: the Diagnostic and Statistical Manual of Mental Disorders—Version 5 (DSM-5), the authoritative and up-to-date (latest revision in 2022) resource that provides a unified classification of mental health and brain-related conditions. DSM-5 offers a common framework and language to define primary psychopathological syndromes and then provides specific criteria to diagnose them.

The manual organizes conditions into chapters that focus on distinct groups of disorders. Neurological disorders, including dementia, are discussed in the Neurocognitive Disorders chapter. Neurocognitive Disorder is a general term that describes decreased cognitive functioning due to a medical disease other than a psychiatric illness. The authors of the Neurocognitive Disorders chapter in DSM-5 included some of the globe's leading experts in geriatric psychiatry, neurology, neuropsychology, and psychiatric research. This group of experts (the Neurocognitive Disorders Work Group) spent five years evaluating the latest advances in scientific knowledge and honing the definitions of neurological conditions. From that effort, they distilled the broad array of neurological difficulties and the various brain illnesses that can produce those difficulties, such as Alzheimer's or cerebrovascular disease, into three primary syndromes, three basic Neurocognitive Disorders (NCDs).

The three basic syndromes or are Delirium, Mild Neurocognitive Disorder, and Major Neurocognitive Disorder.

Delirium is an altered state of consciousness in which the patient is confused, disoriented, and unable to think or remember clearly. It comes rapidly, usually within hours or days, and is treatable, especially if the diagnostician can identify the underlying cause. There is no concern that Trump suffers from delirium.

Nor is there concern that Trump meets the diagnostic criteria for Major Neurocognitive Disorder at the present moment. Major NCD is the syndrome we associate with full-scale dementia, where there is a dramatic loss of capacities that undermines one's ability to live independently.

The syndrome of Mild Neurocognitive Disorder—what we think of as likely early dementia—is the condition that might explain Trump's recent struggles. In Mild NCD, independent living continues, but the person displays moderate decline and signs of struggle in one or more essential areas of functioning.

To determine if Donald Trump displays Mild NCD, we must look at the DSM-5 criteria for this diagnosis. The diagnosis of a Neurocognitive Disorder is all about *the decline* in a critical area of human functioning, referred to as *cognitive domains* in DSM-5. The diagnostician is looking for decline across the following six domains:

Attention

Memory

Language

Executive Functioning

Perceptual-Motor

Social Cognition

The authors of the Neurocognitive Disorder Chapter determined that a decline in *even just one of these domains* warrants consideration of a diagnosis of one of the neurocognitive syndromes. If the decline is "substantial" and the struggle with independent living is significant, the diagnosis of Major NCD (full-blown) dementia is warranted. If the decline is "moderate" and the struggle with independent living is just emerging, a diagnosis of Mild NCD is justified.

If one is suspected to be in the throes of a Neurocognitive Disorder, you would undertake a comprehensive assessment of these domains. The gold standard of such an evaluation would involve administering fine-grained neuropsychological tests in each domain. This is where frustration over Trump's refusal to release details of his medical exams or collaborate in such testing is felt.

However, even without this cooperation, two other sources of potentially relevant information exist: (1) reports from biographers or close observers of Trump and (2) direct observation of his behavior in these domains.

What can we glean from these sources vis-a-vis the six key cognitive domains?

Information from close observers—colleagues, employees, family, friends, and journalists, such as Tony Schwartz, co-author of *The Art of the Deal*—and well-sourced biographies help assess *executive functioning, attention,* and *social cognition.* These domains consist of a broad swath of behavior, much of it occurring off-camera. To get a decent appraisal, one must assess these behaviors over many situations and months, if not years.

We have copious evidence from many insider accounts and biographies that Trump's functioning in these areas is markedly below average. He has a notoriously short attention span, disdains the planning, focus on details, and self-control that comprise executive functioning. He also has a lifelong history of disagreeableness and lack of empathy, qualities at the heart of competent social cognition.

Still, it is hard to argue that Trump's struggles in these areas result from a neurodegenerative disease process. Remember, diagnosing a Neurocognitive Disorder requires the demonstration of *decline* in one or more of the six cognitive domains. A comprehensive review of Trump's biographies reveals persistent deficiencies in attention, executive functioning, and social cognition dating back to childhood and quite prominent in his middle age.

However, thanks to reams of videotape on Trump, we have access to many *behavioral observations* to evaluate for possible cognitive decline, which is particularly relevant for *memory*, *perceptual-motor skills* (how one can navigate the world physically), and *language.*

Trump occasionally mixes up people—Nikki Haley for Nancy Pelosi, mayor Willie Brown for a councilman are recent examples—rather than just names. This confusion can be a sign of cognitive decline in the memory domain. Trump's bent, forward-listing posture, jerking right arm and leg, and arm weakness are also worrisome signs of neurological dysfunction and not just normal aging.[8] However, while there are several red flags of neurological issues for Trump in the areas of memory and perceptual-motor skills, there is not sufficient evidence to give a definitive diagnosis of Neurocognitive Disorder.

We still have one domain to evaluate such a possibility: language. Fortunately, this domain does not require collaboration with Trump because you can execute a detailed, clinically meaningful appraisal directly from speech samples readily available on YouTube. Furthermore, you can zero in on possible decline in the language domain by comparing speech samples from the past to the present.

To measure decline more rigorously, we developed the following checklist of seven specific verbal expressive behaviors linked to neurodegenerative brain illness:

Marker	Definition	Examples
Phonemic Paraphasia	A phonemic paraphasia is an unintended utterance of a word in which the speaker substitutes an inappropriate sound for part of the word. At least half of the word must be said correctly to be considered a phonemic paraphasia.	Examples include saying "dat" instead of "hat" or "tephelone" instead of "telephone."
Semantic Paraphasia	The speaker substitutes an entire word for the intended word.	Saying "rabbit" instead of "cat" or "television" instead of "telephone."
Vocabulary Use	There is a decline in the body of words available and the ability to use them.	Simpler word choices ("thing"), fewer polysyllabic words, over-reliance on superlatives ("greatest")
Disordered Syntax	Disruptions in the arrangement of words and phrases that undermine the creation of well-formed sentences in speech.	More fragmented sentences. Getting words in the wrong order. Less use of proportions and dependent clauses.
Word-Finding Difficulty	A person knows and understands a particular word but has difficulty retrieving and using it in speech.	Filler words such as "um" and "ah." Substitute words with a similar meaning or sound. Word searching behaviors ("piece of paper, um, document, um, um, the Constitution").
Palilalia	The compulsive repetition of one's own words, phrases, or sounds.	"Lady, lady, lady," "it's a mess, it's a mess, it's a mess."
Tangential Speech	The speaker's train of thought wanders and shows a lack of focus.	It drifts off-topic without returning to the original point. It veers into irrelevant topics.

We then applied the checklist to randomly selected speech samples of Trump from his middle age and recent past.[9] Trump displayed shifts in all seven markers. He received ratings of "never" or "rarely" for all markers from the years 1975—2000 versus "moderately" or "frequently" for all markers from the years 2020—present. I also developed a list of seven specific verbal expressive behaviors associated with normal aging, such as speech volume and rate. I applied that checklist to the same Trump speech samples. For a man of his age, Trump displays minimal signs of aging in his verbal expressive behavior.

Thus, Trump shows clinically significant signs of cognitive decline in the lan-

guage domain beyond normal aging.

This conclusion is reinforced by other studies that have examined Trump's language behavior. In "*Trump Wasn't Always So Linguistically Challenged-What Could Explain the Change?*" Begley noted "striking and unmistakable" shifts in his vocabulary level and ability to string sentences together.[10] In "Popular Press Claims Regarding Linguistic Change in President Donald J. Trump," a study that zeroed in on word-finding difficulties, investigators found Trump displayed a "systematic increase in the use of filler words"[11]. The author of a *recent study* that applied a metric of analytic thinking to Trump's contemporary speeches concluded, "I can't tell you how staggering this is. He does not think in a complex way at all."[12] STAT, a media organization focused on health research, asked experts in memory, psychology, and linguistics to compare clips of Trump's speech from 2017 to 2024. They concluded that "Trump's speech included more short sentences, a confused order of words, repetition and extended digressions."[13]

We now have evidence that Donald Trump displays a meaningful decline in language functioning. Language functioning is one of the six key cognitive domains cited in DSM-5, where a moderate decline in functioning is sufficient to trigger a formal diagnosis of Mild Neurocognitive Disorder, a condition associated with underlying brain disease.

The implications of this diagnosis are sobering when one considers the responsibilities of the presidency. First, if Trump shows a meaningful decline in one cognitive domain, troubles will likely emerge in other functioning areas. What might this look like in practical terms? Here are some examples:

· Attention— tasks take longer to complete than previously, and work must be double-checked for errors.

· Executive functioning— more effort to finish multistep projects, trouble resuming an interrupted task, and difficulty organizing and planning.

· Learning and memory— difficulty recalling recent events, relies on reminders and list-making.

· Perceptual-motor skills— relies more heavily on maps or notes for directions.

· Social cognition— less ability to read social cues such as facial expressions, decreased empathy, decreased inhibition.

Second, and most critically, this condition typically progresses to full-scale dementia. How fast? Studies indicate that within just one year, 15 percent[14] or even 20 percent[15] of those with Mild NCD will develop full-scale dementia (Major NCD). That percentage, called the annual conversion rate, applies to successive years, thus increasing the risk of full-scale dementia to over 50% within four years.

Another risk factor for Trump is the fact his father, Fred, was diagnosed with Alzheimer's. Individuals with a first-degree relative, such as a parent, who had Alzheimer's, are more likely to develop the condition—their risk increases by 30 percent[16]. Scientists have identified a gene variant called apolipoprotein4 (APOE4) that increases your risk three times beyond that[17]. Testing for the gene is safe, straightforward, and inexpensive. I could not find anywhere in his reported health records that Trump has taken that genetic test.

Given the evidence of likely neurodegenerative illness, we would like to make a plea to the ex-President:

It might be frightening to undergo a comprehensive neuropsychological workup or genetic testing. Taking such a step is typically considered a personal choice and a protected right for any individual. However, a core value in a democracy is an informed citizenry. Citizens have a right to relevant and meaningful information for those seeking office for positions that affect the general welfare. This duty to inform would include, but not be limited to, considerations of health.

As difficult as it might be, you have a moral duty to inform the public about the distinct possibility that you might be in the beginning stage of a deteriorating neurological disorder. Sir, please do the right thing and collaborate on a comprehensive neuropsychological exam.

Vince Greenwood, Ph.D., is the Founder and Executive Director of the Washington Center for Cognitive Therapy, a mental health practice that specializes in the treatment of anxiety and mood disorders. He has served as a consultant at the National Institute of Mental Health (NIMH) and Johns Hopkins University Hospital. He created Duty to Inform (Dutyto-Inform.org) in 2020, a website devoted to the intersection of psychology and politics.

References

1. Shear, Michael D. (2024). "What Are We Told About the Health of Biden and Trump? They Decide." *New York Times,* April 4. *https://www.nytimes.com/2024/04/04/us/politics/biden-trump-health.html*

2. Aronwald, Bruce. Morristown Medical Group. https://truthsocial.com/@realDonaldTrump/posts/111444920245122377

3. Cameron, Chris, (2023). "Trump Health Report Claims 'Weight Reduction' but Skimps on Specifics." *New York Times,* November 20. *https://www.nytimes.com/2023/11/20/us/politics/trump-medical-report.html*

4. Shear, Michael D. and Altman, Lawrence K. (2018). "Trump Is in 'Excellent Health,' Doctor Says After Exam." *New York Times,* January 12. *https://www.nytimes.com/2018/01/12/us/politics/trump-physical-exam.html*

5. Phelps, Jordyn. (2020). "Trump keeps bragging about acing simple test used to detect mental impairment." *ABCNews.com. https://abcnews.go.com/Politics/trump-bragging-acing-simple-test-detect-mental-impairment/story?id=71945342*

6. Mazza, Ed, (2024). "CNN Doctor Trolls Trump Over 'Dementia' Boast With 1 Simple Sentence." *Yahoo.com. https://www.yahoo.com/news/cnn-doctor-trolls-trump-over-045944368.*

7. Achenbach, Joel and Johnson, Mark, (2024). "What science tells us about Biden, Trump and evaluating an aging brain." *Washington Post,* May 18. https://www.washingtonpost.com/science/2024/05/18/biden-trump-age-cognitive-decline/

8. Cytowic, Richard E. (2020)."We Are Entitled to Ask President Trump for His Brain Scan.*" Psychology Today, October, 2020. https://www.psychologytoday.com/us/blog/the-fallible-mind/202010/we-are-entitled-ask-president-trump-his-brain-scan*

9. Greenwood, Vincent, (2024). "DUTY TO INFORM (PART 1) Does Trump or Biden Display Neurocognitive Disorder? Where We Stand Now." *Medium.com.* https://drvincentgreenwood-89455.medium.com/duty-to-inform-part-1-799a4bdb6829

10. Begley, Sharon, (2017). "Trump wasn't always so linguistically challenged. What could explain the change?" *statnews.com, https://www.statnews.com/2017/05/23/donald-trump-speaking-style-interviews/*

11. Coutanche, Marc and Paulus, John (2018). "An Empirical Analysis of Popular Press Claims Regarding Linguistic Change in President Donald J. Trump." *Frontiers in Psychology,* November 18.

12. Rashid, Hafiz, (2024). "Cognitive Decline? Experts Find Evidence Trump's Mind Is

Slowing." *The New Republic,* August 8.

13. Kilander, Gustaf, (2024). "Experts say Trump's speaking style shows 'potential indications of cognitive decline.'" *Independent,* August 8.

14. Mansoor, David, (2018). *ohsu.edu. https://www.ohsu.edu/sites/default/files/2023-04/IMR23-Thurs-08-Mansoor.pdf*

15. Thaipisuttikul, Papan, Jaikla, Kriengsak, Satthong, Sirikorn, and Wisajun, Pattarabhorn (2022). "Rate of conversion from mild cognitive impairment to dementia in a Thai hospital-based population: A retrospective cohort." *National Library of Medicine, https://www.ncbi.nlm.nih.gov/pmc/articles/PMC8970424/*

16. See "Alzheimer's in the Family," (2019). *Harvard Health Publishing,* January 28. *https://www.health.harvard.edu/mind-and-mood/alzheimers-in-the-family*

17. Bullock, Pam, (2024). "Study Suggests Genetics as a Cause, Not Just a Risk, for Some Alzheimer's." *New York Times*, May 6. *https://www.nytimes.com/2024/05/06/health/alzheimers-cause-gene-apoe4.html*

THE FOUNDERS FEARED A TRUMP, SO WHY COULD THEY NOT PREVENT ONE?

Drew Westen, Ph.D.

The Founders feared that every so often in a democracy, a Donald Trump would emerge. They tried to limit the likelihood, and mitigate the damage, by setting up a democratic republic that not only had checks and balances designed to *reflect* the will of the people but also had procedures that could *undo* the will of the people. Among the latter were electors who could defect, a Congress that could impeach, and Senators originally chosen indirectly by state legislatures, not by "the masses" (then, landowning white men).

They put all these procedures in place because they knew the social contract philosophy that provided the intellectual architecture for the Constitution they devised had a major flaw: Humans are susceptible to demagogues, and demagogues are capable of arousing not only the passions of "the mob" but also what Lincoln might have called the lowest demons of our nature.

None of these philosophers had an answer to this problem. The one who grappled most with it was probably Rousseau, who distinguished between the "general will," the genuine best interest of the people, from the "will of all," the closest approximation to it, namely the outcome of the clash of public and private interests obtained through the democratic process. Most of the time, Rousseau believed the political process would yield a close enough approximation to the collective interest (and if not, with regular elections, the system should be self-correcting). But when the will of all diverged too far from the general will—far enough, as the Founders feared, to bring down the entire edifice of the republic—Rousseau's only answer was a fanciful *deus ex machina*, a divine legislator sent by God to put the people back on the right path.

The Founders would have intuitively recognized Trump, but today, his character is quantifiable. Colleagues and I spent years developing a measure aimed at capturing subtle personality processes seen in clinical practice, from everyday personality "issues" to personality disorders. Unlike models and measures of personality with which readers may be familiar, such as the Myers-Briggs or the Five-Factor-Model, on which people can "diagnose" themselves online, this measure (called the SWAP-II), can only be applied by skilled mental health professionals, as it does not assume that most people have either the expertise or objectivity to score themselves. Because we avoided jargon in constructing the items in the measure, however, the portrait painted by simply examining the highest-scoring items is often readily interpretable by an educated layperson.

In early September 2024, I assessed Trump on the 200-item measure using all available data, based on his voluminous speech and behavior samples and a range of other sources. With the exception of five or six of the 200 items in the instrument, which might have received higher scores if I knew more about how germ-phobic he is or how perverse his sexual fantasies may be (which only a skilled, well-analyzed professional should contemplate, as I suspect it would be like staring at the head of Medusa), I had no trouble producing a personality portrait I believe would correlate strongly with ratings by other trained observers. The following are the 30 items in "most descriptive" range of the instrument:

Profiling Trump

Has an exaggerated sense of self-importance (e.g., feels special, superior, grand, or envied).
Tends to blame own failures or shortcomings on other people or circumstances; attributes his/her difficulties to external factors rather than accepting responsibility for own conduct or choices.
Tends to be deceitful; tends to lie or mislead.
Tends to engage in unlawful or criminal behavior.
When distressed, perception of reality can become grossly impaired (e.g., thinking may seem delusional).
Seeks to be the center of attention.
Has little empathy; seems unable or unwilling to understand or respond to others' needs or feelings.
Tends to become irrational when strong emotions are stirred up; may show a significant decline from customary level of functioning.
Takes advantage of others; has little investment in moral values (e.g., puts own needs first, uses or exploits people with little regard for their feelings or welfare, etc.).
Tends to get into power struggles

Tends to be unreliable and irresponsible (e.g., may fail to meet work obligations or honor financial commitments).
Tends to show reckless disregard for the rights, property, or safety of others.
Seems to treat others primarily as an audience to witness own importance, brilliance, beauty, etc.
Tends to have extreme reactions to perceived slights or criticism (e.g., may react with rage, humiliation, etc.).
Experiences little or no remorse for harm or injury caused to others.
Tends to see own unacceptable feelings or impulses in other people instead of in him/herself.
Tends to feel misunderstood, mistreated, or victimized.
Reasoning processes or perceptual experiences seem odd and idiosyncratic (e.g., may make seemingly arbitrary inferences; may see hidden messages or special meanings in ordinary events).
When upset, has trouble perceiving both positive and negative qualities in the same person at the same time (e.g., may see others in black or white terms, shift suddenly from seeing someone as caring to seeing him/her as malevolent and intentionally hurtful, etc.).
Tends to be hostile toward members of the opposite sex, whether consciously or unconsciously (e.g., may be disparaging or competitive).
Has difficulty making sense of other people's behavior; tends to misunderstand, misinterpret, or be confused by others' actions and reactions.
Has fantasies of unlimited success, power, beauty, talent, brilliance, etc.
Tends to feel s/he is inadequate, inferior, or a failure.
Tends to elicit dislike or animosity in others.
Appears impervious to consequences; seems unable or unwilling to modify behavior in response to threats or negative consequences.
Tends to hold grudges; may dwell on insults or slights for long periods.
Is invested in seeing and portraying self as emotionally strong, untroubled, and emotionally in control, despite clear evidence of underlying insecurity, anxiety, or distress.
Thought processes or speech tend to be circumstantial, vague, rambling, digressive, etc. (e.g., may be unclear whether s/he is being metaphorical or whether thinking is confused or peculiar).
Has little psychological insight into own motives, behavior, etc.
Appears to feel privileged and entitled; expects preferential treatment.

The instrument was designed to assess dimensions of personality, not all forms of psychopathology (e.g., depression, bipolar disorder, anxiety disorders).

In 2008, while Trump was still in an appropriate job, as a reality show host who satisfied his sadism by telling people, "You're Fired," colleagues and I published a study applying statistical procedures to SWAP-II descriptions of hundreds of patients with narcissistic personality disorder to identify subtypes of the disorder (Russ et al., 2008). One of the three that emerged was, in fact, a malignant subtype, at the intersection of narcissistic and psychopathic personality, with significant paranoid features. Trump's profile and the items prototypical of that subtype were virtually indistinguishable, providing a quantified diagnosis of malignant narcissism. The main difference was that Trump's showed more signs of disordered thinking, likely a stronger attribute of authoritarian leaders willing to incarcerate or kill their political opponents than among the malignant narcissists in the range settings from prisons to boardrooms that comprised our patient sample.

Like many of the authors of the first edition of this volume—and comedian Bill Maher, who insisted from the start of Trump's presidency that he would never leave office voluntarily—in the fall of 2020 I predicted a likely coup attempt, based on a combination of Trump's functional deficits (psychological characteristics that should be there but are not, e.g., the capacity for empathy or guilt), psychiatric syndromes (characteristics that should not be there but are, e.g., his unusually large number and severity of personality disorders), and a disturbing pattern of behavior (e.g., discrediting the ballot count in advance, seeking alternative slates of electors, and most ominous, replacing officials in the highest offices in the executive branch, particularly those leading armed forces, with his loyalists) (Westen, 2023).

We should, however, be even more concerned in 2025 if we see Trump Unplugged—from morality, of which he has no concept; reality, of which he has no grasp; and law, to which he now lacks accountability, thanks to some of the unindicted co-conspirators on the Supreme Court. Given the tightness of the race between Trump and first Biden and then Harris, Trump could be elected in 2024, or he could be installed by a judiciary that could take longer this time to hear a larger number of absurd cases objecting to electoral counts, for which the courts should have issued substantial enough Rule 11 (frivolous lawsuit) sanctions against his attorneys in 2020 to deter future such challenges. This time, however, those lawsuits will likely come from dozens of newly elected officials involved in local elections throughout the swing states, who could hold up certification of electors themselves or file legal challenges, some of which would no doubt reach the Supreme Court, at least on appeal. The Court could then either use delay as a decision, as it initially did with Trump's absurd immunity claim, and thus throw selection of the President into the House, it or could issue judgments even more corrupt than its granting Trump immunity for all past and future crimes as President.

I need not spell out the consequences of a second Trump presidency, which he has, himself, spelled out most succinctly in his statement, "I am your retribution," and more comprehensively in the playbook he publicly disavows, *Project 2025*. Either way, however, he has galvanized a movement dominated by grievance, conspiracy theories, and conspiracies; created a cult of personality so bizarre that no one outside it even notices anymore when he makes biblical references to himself, as when, in recently denying a rape allegation, he responded that had he intended to rape a woman, she would not have been "the chosen one," rather than making an equally vulgar claim without the religious grandiosity, such as "the woman I would have chosen to rape"; and united a coalition that promises to be with us for years. That requires us to ask what happened and whether we have learned anything about how to stop it from recurring.

The Founders would certainly have laid the blame for Trump and Trumpism at the feet of a Republican Party that has devolved into pin-striped thuggery, whose leaders have betrayed their country through a paradoxical combination of cowardice in the face of Orange Julius and the masses he can conjure up to invade the Forum, and the single-minded pursuit of power. Both Congressional and judicial Republicans seem, however, to hold the same delusion (for most, in the colloquial sense of the word) that installing a psychopathic, malignant narcissist with full immunity will lead to a power-sharing arrangement. Apparently, they have never read a history of the Soviet Union under Stalin or of any other absolute leader with a similar character structure, or to have noticed what happens to Putin's oligarchs if they serve at the displeasure of the president. Under the Supreme Court's immunity decision, the moment the Supreme Court were to issue an adverse ruling in a second Trump administration, he would simply ignore it or disband the court, just as nothing would prevent him from disbanding a "disobedient" Congress.

A new, illiberal era of Republican politics began in late 2000, when Sandra Day O'Connor, after worrying aloud about a Gore victory because she wanted to retire under a Republican President, cast the deciding vote in Bush v. Gore, which established the precedent that the Supreme Court could pick its own successors. The Court's decision was legally incoherent—as have been many of the decisions of the three of the nine current Justices who served at that time on Bush's legal team in Bush v. Gore—made even more so by the warning label the Court placed on the Pandora's Box it opened, that the decision should somehow not serve as precedent.

Until the two impeachments of Donald Trump, Democrats have repeatedly failed to recognize and prevent attacks on our freedom and to respond with equal, opposite, and appropriate aggression. Had Sandra Day O'Connor been a Democrat who made a Faustian bargain to install a Democrat in the 2000 election, Republicans would have tarred her as a Benedict Arnold who had openly admitted the reason for her breaking her oath to protect and defend the Constitution—her desire to replace a purportedly nonpartisan Justice with a partisan hack—not lionized her for breaking a glass ceiling.

Americans were clamoring for justice, but they got none. Democrats' failures to respond with appropriate and aggressive action only intensified as the dangers escalated in the ensuing years, leading to the attack on the Capital on January 6, 2021.

What the Founders could never have understood about the Insurrection of 2021 was how, as the world's oldest democracy, America could not figure out what some of the youngest democracies had no trouble recognizing when, shortly after the coup attempt in the United Stated, the defeated Presidents of Peru and Brazil did exactly the same thing, after which Germany then uncovered a widespread rightwing plot to overthrow their elected government. They immediately imprisoned or drove the would-be dictators into exile, threw their co-conspirators in parliament in prison, and made clear that anyone who joined them in their conspiracy or spoke in support of the insurrection after they had rounded up the insurrectionists would be bunking up with them that evening and could expect to do so for many years.

What these young democracies did *not* do was to insist that the judicial calendar had nothing to do with the electoral calendar in the face of a coup attempt, so the insurrectionists would be free to run for office again two or four years later. They did not take their time to capture the low-level participants in the coup attempt and eventually prosecute them, while allowing the head and body of the snake to remain free. They did not allow the snake to develop and amplify an alternative narrative, create its own propaganda machines such as "Truth Social" to foster the next coup attempt, or fail to do what any government would do, namely to indict and hold the insurrectionists without bail until they could face trial.

Instead, Garland failed to arrest and detain either the former president or *any* of the congressional, cabinet-level, or other high-ranking leaders of the insurrection, instead putting his obsessional dynamics on display by demanding the application of procedures that would have been inappropriate not only in normal times but especially in the aftermath of a coup attempt. When an assailant attacked Nancy Pelosi's husband, he was immediately held without bond, not released while the police could collect affidavits from the hardware store where he purchased the hammer, statements from friends and neighbors that might speak to his intent, etc.) Garland did not think to read Trump's playbook for overthrowing American Democracy, *Mein Kampf,* in which Hitler explained what he had learned from the first coup, for which he received a brief slap on the wrist: that the way to dismantle a democracy is to get elected and then to use the instruments of the state to dismantle it from within.

So, what needs to be done to keep America safe from enemies from within?

Enough people on both sides of the aisle with the integrity, backbone, and character structure required to enforce the laws that make democracy and freedom possible, who understand that extraordinary times require extraordinary skill in applying the laws and who possess the self-understanding to fight off the twin temptations of complicity or cowardice in the face of fear caused by an organized attack on cherished institutions that protect our freedom. Organized criminal activity aimed at undercutting democracy requires an organized, lawful, aggressive response.

If Trump loses the election but his cultists planted within every branch and level of government challenge the election and have a chance of succeeding, we can only hope President Biden will, with the freedom a corrupt court has provided him to take decisive action without fear of prosecution, act in whatever ways are necessary and possible within the law to prevent the illegitimate use of actions that in themselves would be lawful but when carried out in conspiracy are not. That would not require violating any law but would likely require suspending unwritten norms intended for ordinary times, such as the independence of the Justice Department and the White House, which Trump has promised to end on his first day of office if re-elected or re-installed; firing Merrick Garland; and replacing him with an Attorney General who will warn anyone, including members of the Supreme Court, that this time, any attempt to subvert the will of the people that involves the coordinated action of two or more people will be met with the appropriate application of our criminal statutes including but not limited to conspiracy.

Churchill actually held a more sanguine view than the maxim for which he is often cited, that democracy is the worst form of government except all the others. And he was both right and wrong: Democracy is both the best hope for freedom and the worst form of government except all others. No amount of tinkering with institutions can prevent the occasional perfect storm of a ruthless leader and a coalition of the conniving and cowardly, who lack the foresight to imagine the likely outcome of joining together to bring a malignant charismatic figure to power, especially when those who oppose them respond with obsessional defenses to the conditions under which democracies fail.

To put it another way, sometimes, by an extraordinary, and some might say divine, roll of the historical dice, you get the confluence of a Benjamin Franklin, a George Washington, and a Thomas Jefferson, all living in the same place at the same time, at a moment ripe for a progressive change. And at others, you roll snake eyes, and get a Donald Trump, Ted Cruz, and Josh Hawley. Those are the times that try men's and women's souls.

Drew Westen, Ph.D., is Director of Clinical Psychology at Emory University and is Professor of Psychology and Psychiatry. He is author of The Political Brain: The Role of Emotion in Deciding the Fate of the Nation. For 20 years, he has provided a psychological analysis of political issues, including the influence of non-verbal communication on voter behavior. He has advised or worked as a consultant for presidential, congressional, and state-level candidates, progressive and labor organizations, and Fortune 500 companies. Dr. Westen has written more than 100 scientific papers and two books, including an introductory psychology textbook now in its third edition.

References

Russ, E., Shedler, J., Bradley, R., & Westen, D. (2008). Refining the construct of narcissistic personality disorder: Diagnostic criteria and subtypes. *American Journal of Psychiatry*, *165*(11), 1473-1481.

Westen, D. (2023). TDS Strategy White Paper: All the President's Mental Disorders. *Democratic Strategist*. https://thedemocraticstrategist.org/_white_papers/tds_White_Paper_Drew_Westen.pdf

WHAT MATTERS IN THE TRUMP CANDIDACY

Ellyn Kaschak, Ph.D.

As I and many of my colleagues have noted in writing about Donald Trump, the man is dangerous to other humans of all stripes. Let's consider why that is. Is it because he is clearly a malignant narcissist, interested only in self-promotion, in seizing and holding as much power as possible? Can he be diagnosed with a known and agreed upon mental illness or defect? Even if we permit ourselves to diagnose him, how would that help avoid the havoc that he can and will wreak upon us all? It may help us to predict the inevitable, but then what? It is the "then what?" that I wish to consider here.

My focus is not on mental illness, not cognitive impairment, and not narcissism, but instead on aggression, violence, and danger. Trump is already well-known for assaulting women, denigrating anyone who disagrees with him and elevating grievance to a fine art. Trump harnesses hatred, which he peddles to his followers along with red MAGA hats and the recently profitable white ear bandages.

He is a huckster, a salesman, a purveyor of snake oil. And the marks are all lining up by the millions to purchase these products. "Satisfaction guaranteed. Double your money back if one swallow doesn't take away all your doubts, leaving you feeling comfortable, angry, and self-righteous. Right this way. Learn how to win any argument by ignoring the facts, ridiculing and demeaning your opponent."

"There is no such thing as a discussion. Life is a series of battles that must be won. Winner take all and any effective tactics may and should be used."

The courts, many of whose so-called justices were appointed by Trump during his "gig" as president, having already insulted and assaulted women and their/our rights, have their sights set now on other vulnerable groups, prominent among which are LGBT citizens. If Trump has his way, civil rights will be only a bittersweet memory.

These very same courts have also taken the startling step of providing protection for his proven criminal behavior, by allowing possible impunity for the former president's criminal convictions on some 34 felonies. For the first time in history, the president of the United States could be a convicted criminal.

Should Trump win the election, which is a serious possibility, he will certainly do all he can to dismantle democracy and to turn our country into a dictatorship and himself into president for life.

What could happen if Trump loses the election is almost as alarming as what inevitably will occur if he wins. Chaos, riots, violence, endless grievance. And even if Trump disappears from the scene, his millions of followers will not. Inevitably there will be a Trump Junior, perhaps Junior himself.

Trump is clearly an invention of his own ambition, willing to speak whatever message buys him adulation and power, money, and those cherished votes. Yet he is as much an invention of his constituents as he is of his own mind. He is the living, breathing personification of their values. He is each of them writ large and, in their eyes, can do no wrong. He is probably not wrong when he says he could shoot someone on Fifth Avenue with impunity, certainly in their eyes and increasingly so in the justice system itself.

What can we mental health experts offer at this crucial juncture and what are our obligations? I firmly believe that we must come out of our offices, must not continue only to practice privately and must make visible the connections between the private and the public, the personal and the political. Both professionalism and activism must heed the clarion call. We must help everyone see that delusions are contagious and that we are dealing, in this case, with STDs (Socially Transmitted Diseases).

In my earlier writing in these volumes (Kaschak, 2019), I have offered a tool that I have found useful in conducting therapy, in teaching students who are learning to become peace workers and in doing large scale political work myself. I call this tool the Mattering Map, as it makes visible to all who use it the sometimes-invisible connections between abuse and trauma, between harm and healing, and between all of us who experience these traumas. As a tool that does not pathologize, but unites, that makes visible the personal and the political, the individual and the cultural collective, it can help us to see what is in the margins or kept invisible, the complex causes of STDs that include what are traditionally separated as psychological and cultural influences. What some call meaning, I name the more lusty and passionate term, mattering. To resist, to remain lucid and focused, we must harness the power of what matters in each life. There is no stronger force.

As a tool, it asks each of us to identify the multiple, complex causes of each situation in which we find ourselves individually or collectively.

Gender

Race

Ethnicity

Culture

Language

Class

Ecology

Environment

Physical Health, Biology, Neurology

Family

Interpersonal other than family

Religious-Spiritual

Written and Electronic Media. Level of literacy

Other Institutions, e.g., school, work

Age, Life cycle

Political

Beliefs

Group Memberships

Education

Sexual Orientation

Substance-Use and Abuse

Violence

Finances

Power

Should Trump win the upcoming election and move to make himself president for life, the shock and trauma will be inevitable and collective. Should Trump lose, his minions will most certainly take to the streets in violent protest. Many precincts will refuse to certify the election and Trump himself has already shown that he will not concede.

The Mattering Map has morphed, as it does, in recent days. Trump's own map now introduces another variable to his own complex influences and that variable is time, age. With the changing of his Democratic opponent, Trump becomes the oldest candidate by far. He is 78 years old, only three years younger than Biden and more than eighteen years older than Harris. Should he be elected, he would be 82 by the time he leaves office, should he actually do so. Surely Harris will seize upon this issue to persuade the undecided voters of Trump's vulnerability.

More importantly, she can use Trump's own words to prosecute her case. He has spoken often of the issue of age in regard to Biden. Now his words, in the mouth of his new opponent, come back to bite him. And they will, especially as he himself is providing both ammunition and opportunity. This very week, in his much-touted interview with Elon Musk, he evidenced very clearly that his cognition, his ability to focus and think clearly, is not what it once was. Is age beginning to take its toll? As a psychologist, I must raise this issue, and as a politician, I am sure that Kamala Harris will as well.

We must raise this issue in articles, in interviews and in books such as this one. In doing so, we exercise our ethical responsibility to use our tools in multiple arenas, to educate the public and to work for the common good. And after all, this is what matters most.

Ellyn Uram Kaschak, Ph.D., is one of the founders of feminist psychology. She has been on the faculties of San Jose State University since 1974 and the Universidad Nacional and the University for Peace, both in Costa Rica, and was editor of the Journal of Women and Therapy from 1996 to 2017. Kaschak is the past chair of the Feminist Therapy Institute and a fellow of five APA Divisions. She received awards for her two groundbreaking books, Engendered Lives: A New Psychology of Women's Experience *(1992) and* Sight Unseen: Gender and Race Through Blind Eyes *(2015), as well as numerous other awards, including the Lifetime Achievement Award of the Division on LGBT Issues and the Distinguished Career Award of the Association for Women in Psychology.*

Reference

Kaschak, E. (2019). To Trump, some lives matter. In *The dangerous case of Donald Trump*, (pp. 373-384). New York, NY: St. Martin's Press.

DONALD TRUMP'S WEAPONIZATION OF REALITY

LARRY SANDBERG, M.D.

> In 2023, Trump began talking about using the Department of Justice to arrest his enemies, not because they are guilty of something but because, if he returns to the Presidency, he wants 'retribution.' If he ever succeeds in directing federal courts and law enforcement at his enemies, in combination with a mass trolling campaign, then the blending of the autocratic and democratic would be complete.
>
> Ann Appelbaum, *Autocracy, Inc.*,
> 2024

> Mr. Trump repeatedly revived his false claims of widespread election fraud in 2020 and spun them forward to November... 'That's the one thing—they're [Democrats] great at cheating in elections.'
>
> *New York Times*, August 25, 2024

While Donald Trump lost the 2020 presidential election to Joe Biden, he succeeded in asserting control over the Republican Party and reimagining it in his image. It is now unrecognizable as the party of Abraham Lincoln. Millions of Americans, embracing Donald Trump's lies, harbor the false belief that the 2020 election was stolen and display a deep skepticism about the integrity of our electoral process. The Supreme Court has placed limits on what presidential acts can be prosecuted. A Federal judge, a Trump appointee, has ruled, against all precedent, that a Special Prosecutor has no authority to prosecute Donald Trump for removing documents from the White House. The state election board in Georgia has given election officials the power to delay or refuse certification of the upcoming election. Project 2025, authored by a conservative think tank and former Trump appointees, represents a Republican policy blueprint seen by the historian Heather Cox Richardson as a manifesto for an authoritarian presidency. These are all manifestations of Trumpism, a malignant process that threatens to destroy our democracy. It is a political, social, and cultural movement catalyzed by Donald Trump, who is committed to bending reality to his will using an autocrat's playbook to become one.

Donald Trump's psychology is governed by a transactional, zero-sum mentality that depends upon sowing divisiveness, fear, and mistrust in the service of gaining admiration and power. The judicial, legislative, political, and social climate that exists today affords him enormous power should he win reelection this November. The guardrails of our democracy are being sorely challenged by a man with autocratic leanings who will, quite literally, say and do anything to further his own self-interest. Vulnerable Americans who have been let down by our government and have felt desperate for change have been pawns in Donald Trump's power play. He has denigrated them in private as 'basement dwellers.' Those in our country with a far-right, pro-nationalist, xenophobic, homophobic, misogynistic agenda who seek to erode our democracy have used Donald Trump to further their own agenda: a marriage of convenience, giving him the love, admiration, and power he craves in exchange for policies that, at their core, are anti-democratic and deeply unpopular. Defeating Donald Trump is an essential step towards reclaiming our democracy and eradicating the existential threat posed by him.

Donald Trump is anything but subtle. His psychology, as evidenced by his words and actions, is on clear display. I will focus on Trump's problematic relationship with reality and his effort to misuse reality to gain power and control, manipulate others, and manage a fragile self-esteem that feels under constant threat. This is one consideration, among many, that makes him unfit for the office of the Presidency and a danger to our country and the world order.

Reality testing is a crucial capacity for mental health. It can be disrupted in many kinds of conditions. Regardless, it is a foundational aspect of mental functioning that allows us to see reality as it is—undistorted by our wishes, needs, or emotions. Good reality testing is essential for objectivity and is a prerequisite for effective problem-solving. If you cannot see reality for what it is, if you cannot accept reality, you cannot effectively problem solve. For some individuals, reality testing is challenged when facing inevitable painful aspects of life. A strong sense of self and good self-esteem support us during these moments. We all face loss, disappointment, failure, and criticism. Donald Trump repeatedly reveals himself incapable of adequately coping with these realities. His perception of reality must be updated to a more palatable, albeit highly problematic, 'truth.'

Examples abound daily that illustrate this vulnerability. Kamala Harris did not have a larger crowd at her rally than he did at his. She lied by using artificial intelligence. In an interview with Black journalists, it is not Trump who is being hostile and attacking; it is the journalists asking him hard questions who are hostile. When confronted with the radical nature of Project 2025, he claims to know nothing about it. Yet this roadmap involved contributions by over 100 people in Trump's Administration. Daniel Patrick Moynihan, the late Senator from New York, famously said, 'You are entitled to your own opinion, but you are not entitled to your own facts.' Not so with Donald Trump. His 'facts' are fluid, governed by his emotional needs. The 2020 election cycle powerfully demonstrates this tendency and is a harbinger of what lies ahead.

Donald Trump lost the 2020 election and claimed, and continues to claim that the election was stolen. He cannot accept that he lost because Americans preferred Joe Biden. No. He was mistreated, victimized, and wronged. He conjured a theory, a conspiracy, that soothed his ego while also enraging him. And he infected his followers with this belief by actively encouraging them to believe this falsity and feel aggrieved and, also, enraged. He used his position of power, authority, and trust to indoctrinate millions of Americans with a lie. This culminated in the attack on the Capital, where many of the participants, believing Trump's conspiracy theory, were convinced they were acting patriotically. To be clear—Trump's incapacity to accept defeat compelled him to generate a conspiracy theory and incite his followers to break the law. His own legal troubles tied to his defeat further evidence the extreme steps he will take if reality does not conform to his emotional needs.

Two points of clarification. An individual cannot deny a reality he does not, on some level, know to be true. As with Lady Macbeth ('methinks the lady doth protest too much'), the intensity with which he protests reflects his awareness of what he is facing. In this respect, Donald Trump both knows and does not know reality. He argues that the 2020 election was stolen, but news reports indicate he has acknowledged having lost. More pernicious is his effort to create an alternative reality in the minds of others to garner their support. In this dynamic state, Trump is a victim but also not a victim. He bends reality so that he is standing up and fighting for those who are being wronged, disenfranchised. His real 'strength' is in manipulating his followers to believe he is looking out

51

for them when, in reality, he is using them to fight his battle. This is what distinguishes a 'sore loser' from a dangerous sore loser. The denial, distortion, persistent attack, and ultimate destruction of consensual reality are dictatorial.

So here in 2024, Trump is once again constructing a false narrative, campaigning based on a lie, utilizing a strategy suited to dictators, not a politician in a democratic society. Donald Trump acts as if he knows and can predict the future with certainty. He knows if the election is fair and free, that he will win. He knows if he loses that the election will be stolen. Once again, the victim. And, if the election is stolen then, of course, it is an outcome he cannot accept. And he must fight for his supporters who must fight for truth and justice.

We have seen this show before, and we know how it ends. Donald Trump is distorting and attempting to weaponize reality. He is intentionally sowing doubts and mistrust amongst his followers as to the integrity of our voting system. It is 2020 all over again. He is threatening to fight the results of the 2024 election if they do not suit him and to potentially interfere with the peaceful transfer of power. Using a page out of an autocratic playbook, he argues and tries to convince his supporters that they are the real victims, they are the ones being cheated. Sowing dissension, disunity, and polarization to bend reality and soothe his ego.

The current state of the Republican Party foreshadows what a Trump presidency in 2024 would bring. When ultimate power is achieved, love and admiration are no longer necessary; one rules by fear. Republicans who despised Trump and all that he represented now sing his praises. They have made a pact with the devil, pinning their own career ambitions on a man with no moral compass or clear values whose transactional nature permeates all his relationships, including his fluid relationship with reality. Defeating Donald Trump is an essential step in restoring health to the Republican Party and our two-party system. Project 2025 gives us reason to fear that Trump would attempt to accomplish in our country what he has wrought within the Republican Party.

How do we move forward? I think that we must recognize the seductive power of Donald Trump's paranoid vision of the world. We must empathize with the real-life suffering of so many Americans who, in their state of desperation with worsening social and economic inequality, were drawn to a demagogue. Regardless of our party affiliation, regardless of where we stand on issues, we must support leaders who appreciate and respect the complexity of the world, who avoid black-and-white thinking and demonization. We need leaders to lead, not to function as cult figures, and not to act as one.

We need leaders who encourage us to fight for what we believe in, not to fight with one another. We need the fear so many of us experience to mobilize us, not paralyze us, as we step forward and take responsibility for doing what we can, what we must, to ensure our democracy survives.

Larry Sandberg, M.D., is a clinical associate professor of psychiatry at Weill-Cornell Medical College and on the teaching faculty at Columbia University Center for Psychoanalytic Training and Research. He has written on combining different therapeutic modalities to optimize clinical outcomes and on the relationship between neuroscience and psychotherapy. In 2018, he interviewed Dr. Bandy Lee for the Journal of Psychodynamic Psychiatry *to address the ethical role and responsibility of psychiatrists to comment on public figures. He is the author of several influential letters in the* New York Times. *He is in private practice in New York City.*

ON THE ORIGIN AND SPREAD OF DONALD TRUMP'S CONSPIRACY CLAIM THAT THE DEMOCRATS STOLE THE ELECTION

HANS WERBIK, PH.D.

To examine whether Trump's conspiracy narrative that Democrats stole votes from him in the 2020 presidential election is a lie—in everyday language, this conspiracy narrative is called the "Big Lie"— we need to look at Trump's motivation.

Tony Schwartz, who wrote the book "The Art of the Deal" together with Trump and therefore knows Trump well personally, writes about him:

"Instead, Trump grew up fighting for his life and taking no prisoners. In countless conversations, he made clear to me that he treated every encounter as a contest he had to win, because the only other option from his perspective was to lose, and that was the equivalent of obliteration. Many of the deals in the 'The Art of the Deal' were massive failures—among them the casinos he owned and the launch of a league to rival the National Football League—but Trump had me describe each of them as a huge success. ... What's clear is that he has spent his life seeking to dominate others, whatever that requires and whatever collateral damage it creates along the way. A key part of that story is that facts are whatever Trump deems them to be on any given day. ... His aim is never accuracy; it's domination. Trump's need for unquestioning praise and flattery also helps to explain his hostility to democracy and to a free press—both of which thrive on open dissent."[1]

In summary, one can say about Trump's motivation: he cannot stand failure. Due to his extreme narcissism and his strong striving for dominance, he has to reinterpret failures in such a way that the result corresponds to his narcissism and his striving for dominance. The inevitable consequence is a distortion of his perception of reality and a severe impairment of judgment.

An unbiased evaluator can observe this consequence in the fact that Trump keeps exaggerating his assertion: in an interview, he claimed that the result of the 2020 presidential election is "the greatest fraud in the history of our country from an electoral standpoint."[2]

In a speech in Arizona in July of 2021, he claimed, "The radical left Democrat communist party rigged and sold the election."[3]

Applying this to Trump's conspiracy narrative, we can conclude: as a result of his personality, Trump was unable to acknowledge Joe Biden's election victory. The thought that Biden, and not he, won the election was unbearable. Therefore, he invented the claim that the Democrats had stolen votes from him. Trump's inner convictions are that he actually won the election. Therefore, there is no contradiction between Donald Trump's claim and his inner convictions. There are also no ulterior motives since his intention to stay in power is obvious.

These arguments imply that Trump's conspiracy narrative is no lie. But what is it then?

We will find an answer to this question by examining Trump's freedom of action. Is Trump free to act with regard to his claim? Trump gives off the impression that he actually doesn't have any freedom to act anymore with regard to this issue—he seems compelled to repeat his claim every chance he gets; he keeps having to make it sound more drastic every time; he has to assert his claim no matter what. He appears like a man driven by his thirst for dominance and his narcissism. If this is true, then his claim is a pathological misstatement.

There is an episode which confirms this impression of Trump as a man driven by a thirst for dominance and narcissism:

On June 3, 2021, Alex Henderson writes on Alternet: "Earlier this week, the New York Times' Maggie Haberman reported that Donald Trump expects to be "reinstated" as President by August. ... But conservative journalist Charles C.W. Cooke, in an article for the National Review, reported that Haberman was not fear-mongering and that Trump really does believe he will be returning to the Oval Office this summer. 'Haberman's reporting was correct,' Cooke writes, 'I can attest, from speaking to an array of different sources, that Donald Trump does indeed believe quite genuinely that he ... will be 'reinstated' to office this summer after 'audits' of the 2020 elections in Arizona, Georgia and a handful of other states have been completed. I can attest, too, that Trump is trying hard to recruit journalists, politicians and other influential figures to promulgate this belief—not as a fundraising tool or an infantile bit of trolling or a trial balloon, but as a fact. The scale of Trump's delusion is quite startling,' Cooke writes. '... 'It is a rejection of reality, a rejection of law, and, ultimately, a rejection of the entire system of American government. There is no Reinstatement Clause within the Unites States Constitution.' Cooke notes that the 'cold, hard neutral facts' show that the 2020 election was 'absolutely not' stolen as Trump claims...."[4]

Moreover, the fact that Donald Trump never presented any evidence or proof to corroborate his claim should not be neglected. For this reason, the Supreme Court rejected Trump's election challenge cases.

Regarding Trump's way of dealing with facts, it is shockingly similar to Hitler's and Stalin's. By pointing this out, I am obviously not saying that Trump could be compared with Hitler or Stalin on the whole. In "The Origins of Totalitarianism", the famous Jewish philosopher Hannah Arendt wrote: "Konrad Heiden, Der Fuehrer: Hitler´s Rise to Power, Boston 1944, underlines Hitler´s 'phenomenal untruthfulness', 'the lack of demonstrable reality in nearly all his utterances', his indifference to facts which he does not regard as vitally important' (pp.368,374)—In almost identical terms, Krushchev described 'Stalin´s reluctance to consider life´s realities' and his indifference to 'the real state of affairs'.... Stalin´s opinion of the importance of facts is best expressed in his periodic revisions of Russian history."[5]

Eric Alterman outlines Donald Trump's lying nature in detail in his book "Lying in State".[6]

During his speech in Arizona, Trump claimed: "I'm the one trying to save American democracy". This statement is by no means credible. It is the nature of democracy for the minority to accept the decision of the majority. And this is precisely what Trump refuses to do.

The attempt to override a democratic majority decision by a mass demonstration and subsequent storming of the Capitol on January 6, 2021 was an attempt at a coup d'état from above, so it was anything but democratic.

One possible interpretation of Trump's statement is that he wants a democracy without the Democrats. Against this, one can only say with Rosa Luxemburg: "Freedom is always the freedom of dissenters."

The conduct he demands from his supporters—one must not contradict him—is profoundly undemocratic. Dissent is an element of democracy.

Let's move on to the prevalence of Trump's conspiracy narrative among American citizens, especially Republican voters.

According to 2021 polls, two-thirds of Republican voters believe the 2020 presidential election was rigged by Democrats. Taking into consideration how deeply divided American society is, the cognition among Republicans that "Democrats are bad, they will stop at nothing" plays into this. As the Washington Post[7] reported on June 24, 2021, wealthy Americans are funding propaganda resources (movies, rallies) to further spread Trump's conspiracy narrative that Democrats stole votes from him. Apparently, wealthy Americans are so afraid of a property tax that they will use any means to weaken the Democrats.

By constantly repeating Trump's claim and spreading it widely, the collateral damage is the destruction of the confidence of millions of Americans in the reliability of the democratic institution of elections.

In the Republican-ruled state of Texas, an attempt is being made to make elections acceptable to Republican voters again by introducing a new election law. Going along with the principle of "democracy, but preferably without the Democrats," new, stricter rules (restricting absentee voting, limiting the opening hours of polling places) will effectively exclude groups of voters who usually vote for the Democratic Party from exercising their right to vote.

If two-thirds of Republican voters believe Donald Trump's conspiracy narrative, the question arises as to why these voters believe anything Trump says. One possible answer is that Trump has been a credible president from the perspective of Republican voters. His campaign promises (e.g., building a wall on the border with Mexico, withdrawing U.S. troops from Afghanistan) and his "America first" policies were very attractive to Republicans. He really made an effort to keep his campaign promises. Republican voters have generalized Trump's credibility and applied it to the new situation. Republican voters are on average less educated than Democratic voters and therefore less accustomed to critical thinking. Thus, hardly anyone wonders how exactly votes could have been stolen when the votes were counted by hand (in some cases several times) and how the election officials and the numerous election observers could have been deceived. The approval of Republican voters is facilitated by the fact that Trump does not provide any direction in terms of content and politics. His political program is limited to anti-communism and ethnocentrism. Trump's striving for dominance is matched by the Republican Party's subordination to him. Complementarily, authoritarian personalities as described by Theodor Adorno[8] are attracted. By this I do not intend to say that all Republicans are authoritarian personalities; I am merely asserting a tendency. Loyalty to Trump is a very high value within the Republican Party. Subordination to the leader is a key characteristic of fascist movements. Whether the Trump movement within the Republican Party is a fascist movement cannot be said for certain because the characteristic of anti-Semitism that is essential to fascist movements is missing. Only individual statements by Trump supporters are anti-Semitic, for example, by Republican Representative Marjorie Taylor Green, who has claimed that the wildfires in California were caused by a space laser funded by wealthy Jews with connections to the Democrats.[9] As for Trump himself, he has never distanced himself from fascist groups that support him. Instead, he has called them patriots.

Among the highly problematic Trump supporters is the QAnon cult. QAnon followers believe the world is ruled by a Satanic elite that sexually abuses and kills young children. Trump is the savior (messiah) for the QAnon sect and is worshipped by them. Through a "storm," QAnon followers believe, the Satanic elite will be swept away and Trump will be reinstated as president of the United States.

Republican Rep. Marjorie Taylor Green, who holds Trump in the highest esteem, was a QAnon follower for some time. According to 2021 polls, 23 percent of Republican voters are QAnon supporters.[10] Trump has never distanced himself from QAnon, but enjoys the adoration that satisfies his narcissism.

Finally, we need to shed a light on Trump's emotional relationship with his supporters. It is a symbiotic-libidinous relationship. Trump needs cheering supporters to satisfy his narcissism; his supporters feel especially respected and loved because of the special attention Trump pays to them. Therefore, "die-hard" Trump supporters cannot be convinced with rational arguments that Biden won the 2020 presidential election and that Trump's claim is false.

The "collateral damage" of Trump's conspiracy narrative includes very dangerous developments. Republican Congressman Madison Cawthorn declared at a pro-Trump meeting in North Carolina: "If our election systems continue to be rigged and continue to be stolen, then it's gonna lead to one place and that's bloodshed."[11]

All in all, as American psychiatrist Bandy Lee says, Donald Trump is a dangerous personality.

Hans Werbik, Ph.D., was born on February 27, 1941 in Hollabrunn, Austria. From 1959 to 1963, he studied psychology, philosophy and musicology at the University of Vienna and received his doctorate in 1963. He then worked as a research assistant at the University of Tübingen, where he completed his habilitation in 1969 with a thesis on the information content and emotional effect of music. In 1970, he moved to the University of Erlangen-Nuremberg, where he was appointed full professor in 1973. He died on December 20, 2021. Hans Werbik is considered one of the founders of German cultural psychology.

References

Schwartz, Tony (2019): I Wrote the Art of the Deal with Donald Trump: His Self-Sabotage is Rooted in His past, In: Lee, Bandy (ed.): The Dangerous Case of Donald Trump. New York: St. Martin's Press, p. 65-67.

Donald Trump: Phone interview with Maria Bartiromo of Fox Business during the show "Sunday Morning Futures" aired on Fox News on 11/29/2020.

Donald Trump: Speech in Arizona on 7/24/2021. https://www.rev.com/blog/transcripts/donald-trump-phoenix-arizona-rally-speech-transcript-july-24.

Hederson, Alex: He's a madman: Conservative confirms Trump believes the 'delusion' he will be reinstalled as president. Alter Net, June 03, 2021.

Arendt, Hannah (2017/1951): The Origins of Totalitarianism. Penguin Random House UK, p. 458, footnote 27.

Eric Alterman (2020): Lying in State. Why presidents lie - and why Trump is worse. New York: Hachette Book Group.

Rosalind S. Helderman, Emma Brown, Tom Hamburger and Josh Dawsey, 24 June 2021: 'Inside the shadow reality world' promotes the lie that the presidential election was stolen. Wealthy allies of former president Donald Trump have spent millions on films, rallies and other efforts to tout falsehoods about the 2020 vote. Washington Post.

Adorno, Theodor W. (2020/1950): Studien zum autoritären Charakter (The authoritarian personality). Frankfurt: Suhrkamp.

Christian Zaschke: Im Bann des Götzen, Süddeutsche Zeitung am 05.02.2021.

Ariel Edwards-Levy CNN, May 28, 2021: Polls find most Republicans say 2020 election was stolen and roughly one quarter embrace QAnon conspiracies. https://edition.cnn.com/2021/05/28/politics/poll-qanon-election-conspiracies/index.html.

Peter H. Lewis, September 2, 2021: "It's going to lead to one place…bloodshed" What Madison Cawthorn said to supporters. https://avlwatchdog.org/its-going-to-lead-to-one-place-bloodshed-what-madison-cawthorn-said-to-supporters/

PART 2
EROS
(LIFE IMPULSE)

DONNY AND BIBI
Mirroring and Twinship
AVNER FALK, PH.D.

Donald Trump's mother called him "Donny." Binyamin Netanyahu's called him "Bibi." While Americans do not refer to Trump by his childhood name, Israelis commonly refer to their prime minister by his.

In psychopolitical terms, Trump is a "mirror-hungry" leader who needs his followers to mirror himself to him, including his thoughts, feelings, and self-image.[1] He likes people who give him the "mirroring" of himself that he is hungry for. They satisfy his deep emotional need and make him happy.

On Monday, March 25, 2019, upon his return from his Shangri-La at Mar-a-Lago to Washington, the day after his attorney general "cleared" him of collusion with the Russians in the 2016 election, the seventy-two-year-old U.S. President Donald Trump received his chief foreign admirer, the sixty-nine-year-old Israeli prime minister Bibi Netanyahu, who had come to see Trump two weeks before a general election in Israel that would decide his political future.

While there are obvious differences between Donny and Bibi in origins, upbringing, and culture, the two men are political and psychological twins. Both had tyrannical fathers who preferred their elder brothers. Both had cold, distant, and infantilizing mothers. Like Trump, Bibi is paranoid and narcissistic.[2]

Like Trump, Bibi is a nationalist, right-wing leader who thrives on incitement, fear, and hate. Like Trump, Bibi acts as if he is entitled to do whatever he likes and is above the law. Like Trump, he has broken the law many times and had been investigated by his country's law-enforcement authorities for his crimes; the Israeli attorney general had announced that he would indict Netanyahu on charges of bribery and breach of public trust.[3]

Three former commanders-in-chief of the Israeli defense forces had formed a new political party called *Blue and White* to oppose Bibi in the upcoming elections. Like Trump's political future, Bibi's hangs in the balance. Both men face removal from office, if not jail terms. Like Trump, Bibi is a greedy, self-destructive narcissistic leader who exploits others for his own needs and has little empathy for their pain. Both of them get their narcissistic pleasure from defeating others and putting them down, rather than from lifting them to their own level.

Nations and countries are products of collective psychology. The psychoanalyst Erik Erikson[5] called them "pseudo-species,"[5] his colleague Vamık Volkan studied their "large-group psychology," and the political scientist Benedict Anderson[6] called them "imagined communities."[7] Trump led the world's wealthiest and mightiest nation; Bibi led one of the world's tiniest countries, albeit one with a special place in world history, a strong military, and nuclear weapons.

But the size of their respective countries did not matter. What did matter to Donny and Bibi was their mutual mirroring and "twinship" relationship. The two leaders used one another to fight their investigators and advance their political careers.[8] With Donald Trump, flattery gets you everywhere. "Bibi," who knew that, who had spent a good part of his younger life in the United States, and who spoke English fluently, fed Trump's narcissism by dressing like him, agreeing with him on everything and heaping praise on him.

The U.S. president was delighted. Having moved his embassy to the contested Israeli capital of Jerusalem the year before, Trump now gave Bibi another huge political gift by formally recognizing the formerly-Syrian Golan Heights, which Israel had occupied since 1967 and annexed in 1981, as an integral part of Israel. Among the Israeli nationalists, this could help Bibi win the election, giving him yet another term as prime minister,[9] but it could also further weaken U.S. Democratic support for Israel, which had been steadily decreasing.[10]

Both Trump and Netanyahu were short-sighted. Their political gains from their mutual-admiration society were short-lived. In the longer term, both these dangerous, malignantly-narcissistic leaders could bring about their own personal destruction, if not that of their countries and the entire world.

Avner Falk, Ph.D., was born in British Palestine, now Israel, in 1943. He obtained his B. Soc. Sc. from the Hebrew University of Jerusalem and his Ph.D. in clinical psychology from Washington University in St. Louis, Missouri. He returned to Israel to teach and engage in private practice. He published psychoanalytic biographies of Moshe Dayan, David Ben-Gurion, Theodor Herzl, Napoleon, Barack Obama, and S. Y. Agnon. His Fratricide in the Holy Land: A Psychoanalytic View of the Arab-Israeli Conflict *won an Outstanding Academic Title Award. A revised edition of his* Franks and Saracens: Reality and Fantasy in the Crusades *is forthcoming.*

References

Jerrold M. Post, "The Charismatic Leader-Follower Relationship and Trump's Base," in Bandy X. Lee (Ed.), The Dangerous Case of Donald Trump: 37 Psychiatrists and Mental Health Experts Assess a President—Updated and Expanded with New Essays, New York, Thomas Dunne Books, 2019, pp. 385-396.

Shaul Kimhi, "The psychological profile of Benjamin Netanyahu using behavior analysis," in Ofer Feldman & Linda O. Valenty (Eds.), Profiling Political Leaders: Cross-Cultural Studies of Personality and Behavior, Westport, Connecticut, Praeger, 2001, pp. 149-164.

Yonah Jeremy Bob, "Mandelblit announces intent to indict Benjamin Netanyahu for bribery," in The Jerusalem Post, March 1, 2019.

Erik Homburger Erikson (1902-1994), German-American psychoanalyst, biographer of Martin Luther and Mahatma Gandhi, best known for his theory on the stages of the human "life cycle" and for the notion of "identity crisis".

Erik H. Erikson, "Pseudospeciation in the Nuclear Age," in Political Psychology, vol. 6, no. 2, June 1985, pp. 213-217.

Benedict Richard O'Gorman Anderson (1936-2015), British-Irish-American political scientist and historian who studied the origins of nationalism.

Benedict Anderson, Imagined Communities: Reflections on the Origin and Spread of Nationalism, Revised edition, London and New York, Verso, 2006.

Deirdre Shesgreen, "Trump-Netanyahu: How two leaders reap political rewards from their cozy relationship," in USA Today, March 25, 2019.

Netanyahu had "served" as PM of Israel from 1996 to 1999 and from 2009 to 2019.

Ishaan Tharoor, "Trump and Netanyahu keep on colluding," in The Washington Post, March 26, 2019.

TRUMP AND VANCE
From Different Isolation to
Shared Dangerousness

Edwin B. Fisher, Ph.D.

Isolation is a key feature among the many things that make Donald Trump dangerous. I described this in *The Dangerous Case of Donald Trump: 27 Psychiatrists and Mental Health Experts Assess a President* (Fisher, 2017) and predicted its narrowing as the demands for confirmation and harsh expulsion of perceived traitors winnowed the coterie to loyalists. This has become apparent such as in the departure several years ago of Hope Hicks, his previously highly-trusted assistant, or, more recently, in the absence of former cabinet members and former Vice President Mike Pence from the 2024 Republican National Convention, and the number of former Trump administration appointees now signing statements against his candidacy.

Now comes J.D. Vance. The circumstances of *Hillbilly Elegy* (Vance, 2016) could not be more unlike the real estate empire in which Trump was raised. But the isolation is similarly profound and, in spite of great differences in family background, it similarly grows into alienation, othering of opponents, valuing of aggression, and consequent danger.

Isolation

Trump has lived an isolation of privilege, growing up the son of a wealthy real estate developer who imposed the importance of defeating and winning. His niece, Mary Trump, described the individual isolation within the family (Trump, 2020). One of the most striking examples was Donald's father, Fred Trump (her grandfather) in his response to his wife's emergency hysterectomy during which she came close to death. According

67

to Mary Trump's family history, he told his daughter, "Go to school tomorrow. I'll call you if there's any change." Mary Trump continues, "She understood the implication: I will call you if your mother dies" (Trump, 2020).

Throughout his life, Trump has elaborated a transactional, ruthless approach to others such as in oft-documented stiffing of contractors or the many cases of throwing under the bus former colleagues who earn his displeasure. By making all others objects, by making his the only subjectivity, makes himself alone. He then seeks out mirrors of his sense of who he is in blends of stardom, protection, and refuge, always however being "The Donald" in Bedminster and *Mar a Lago*. The psychological importance of this to him is suggested by the retained trappings of the White House as backdrop.

In contrast to the coldness within the Trump household, Vance details a culture of extreme closeness within families but closeness in fierce suspicion and defiance of those outside them. Proudly referring to himself and his family as "hillbillies," he sees their ways as separated from the middle class, white, relatively privileged world around them. There is a pride in this. Vance writes in *Hillbilly Elegy*, "Why, I'd ask my grandma ... did everyone stop for the passing hearse? Because, honey, we're hill people. And we respect our dead" (Vance, 2016).

Adding another dimension, Vance notes:

I knew even as a child that there were two separate sets of mores and social pressures. My grandparents embodied one type: old-fashioned, quietly faithful, self-reliant, hardworking. My mother and, increasingly, the entire neighborhood embodied another: consumerist, isolated, angry, distrustful (Vance, 2016).

Vance's sense of difference from others was apparent in his acceptance speech for the vice-presidential nomination at the Republican Convention. He asserted that America "is not just an idea. It is a group of people with a shared history and a common future. It is, in short, a nation," a "homeland" (Bouie, 2024). With its echo of fascist rhetoric, the unstated is clear: there are those—we—who are in the homeland, and those, they, who are not.

Isolation, Grievance, Othering

For decades, the study of violence and aggression has noted the role of dehumanizing the other (Bandura & Walters, 1959). In tight complement to isolation—the "them" to our "us"—othering is a recurrent theme in *Hillbilly Elegy:*

Some people may conclude that I come from a clan of lunatics. But the stories made me feel like hillbilly royalty, because these were classic good-versus-evil stories, and my people were on the right side. My people were extreme, but extreme in the service of something—defending a sister's honor or ensuring that a criminal paid for his crimes (Vance, 2016).

Othering continues as a frequent trope of Vance, including the recent talk of "childless cat women" and then aggressively defending the rhetoric—"If people can't take a joke"—followed by a sitting US Senator saying of the sitting Vice President: "Kamala Harris can go to hell" (Yilek, 2024).

With Trump, the othering is prominent in the talk of "losers," "suckers," and so many more that have become familiar. Trump has been extremely talented at finding the description that "takes" in taking down an opponent, e.g., "Little Marco" and "Low-Energy Jeb." (His apparent failure to equal these in struggling to find a pejorative for Ron DeSantis or, now, Kamala Harris—other than reversion to schoolyard mispronunciation—is perhaps indicative of cognitive changes beyond the scope of this essay.)

Teaching and Valuing Aggression

Vance's dedication to *Hillbilly Elegy* (2016), published when he was 32, is to his grandparents who raised him through much of his childhood: "For Mamaw and Papaw, my very own hillbilly terminators." There follows an enormous number of examples of attacks in response to slights, continuing the theme of isolation, othering, aggression:

- An uncle took exception to being told by a delivery driver to, "Off-load this now, you son of a bitch,"—the exception being the implication that his mother was a bitch. When the driver refused to recant, "Uncle Pet did what any rational business owner would do: He pulled the man from his truck, beat him unconscious, and ran an electric saw up and down his body."
- When she was 12, Mamaw shot a man trying to steal the family's cow. "According to family lore ... The would-be thief could barely crawl, so Mamaw approached him, raised the business end of her rifle to the man's head, and prepared to finish the job. Luckily for him, Uncle Pet intervened. Mamaw's first confirmed

kill would have to wait for another day."

- "Or there was that day when Uncle Teaberry overheard a young man state a desire to 'eat her panties,' a reference to his sister's (my Mamaw's) undergarments. Uncle Teaberry drove home, retrieved a pair of Mamaw's underwear, and forced the young man—at knifepoint—to consume the clothing."
- "Mamaw told Papaw ... that if he ever came home drunk again, she'd kill him. A week later, he came home drunk again and fell asleep on the couch. Mamaw, never one to tell a lie, calmly retrieved a gasoline canister from the garage, poured it all over her husband, lit a match, and dropped it on his chest ... Miraculously, Papaw survived the episode with only mild burns" (Vance, 2016).

Vance reflects on these and other examples as follows:

The Blanton men [Mamaw's side], like the tomboy Blanton sister whom I called Mamaw, were enforcers of hillbilly justice, and to me, that was the very best kind (Vance, 2016).

Toward the end of *Hillbilly Elegy,* Vance returns to this endorsement, "I believe we hillbillies are the toughest goddamned people on this earth. We take an electric saw to the hide of those who insult our mother. We make young men consume cotton undergarments to protect a sister's honor (Vance, 2016)."

Consider how, in the last page of your memoir, in an Afterword, you might end this sentence of appreciation for the grandmother who raised you, "I knew that a sick old woman could be a mother, a caretaker, a protector, an ass chewer, a gun shooter, a grandmother, and I knew—and I needed to know it—that that woman, my Mamaw, _____." How would you finish this sentence? Vance chose "...my Mamaw would kill for me if she had to" (Vance, 2016).

Donald Trump or his father have probably never carried a shotgun or wielded a handgun in a confrontation or lifted a chainsaw, if at all, surely not in anger. The modes of aggression are varied. But the themes and harms begin to converge. In Mary Trump's telling, Fred Trump's household may have been devoid of almost any caring or love, but was dominated by overwhelming and unceasing pressure, ruthlessly never to be a loser. As both Donald Trump and Melania Trump have articulated in recent years, "When you attack him, he will punch back 10 times harder," (Trump, 2020). But the realities of family wealth saw the punching, domination, and winning more in the coinage of creditors dismissed or business deals exploited, as well as sexual assault, housing discrimination, or this year's 34 convictions for business fraud and pay-offs to make inconvenient things or people go away.

Some of Trump's aggression may be merely transactional, just business. Through this, however, a total absorption in self and disregard for others has been widely noted. There is also gratuitous cruelty revealed in almost trivial acts such as not allowing devout Sean Spicer to join an audience with the Pope during Trump's first international trip as president (Gaffey, 2017). The January 6th Committee hearings documented his enjoying the assault on the Capitol from his private dining room, in spite of the clearly emerging harm to many, and adamantly refusing to do anything to stop it. Breathtaking are the cruelty in exploiting the rioters, one of whom was killed and many of whom were injured and/or have done jail time, along with his dismissal of threats to his Vice President with, "he deserved it."

Perhaps Fred Trump's world of New York real estate and Mamaw's world of hillbillies come closest to converging in praise of violence or aggression. Examples include:

- Mamaw's grandfather got away with killing a member of a feuding, rival family. Vance says that, when he read about this in the New York Times, "I felt one emotion above all the rest: pride. It's unlikely that any other ancestor of mine has ever appeared in The New York Times. Even if they had, I doubt that any deed would make me as proud as a successful feud."
- After Vance's sister was jilted, he describes seeing her ex-boyfriend, "walking past our house one day. He had five years and about thirty-five pounds on me ... [and] proceeded to pound the shit out of me. I ran to Mamaw's house for some first aid, crying and a little bloody. She just smiled at me. 'You did good, honey. You did real good.'"
- Following Vance's successful challenge, a school bully, "... was alternately coughing and trying to catch his breath. He even spit up a small amount of blood ... Mamaw found out about the fight directly from me and praised me for doing something really good."
- After Vance's mother fought another mother following exchanged insults at, "one of my second-grade football games, ... I asked Mom what happened, and she replied only, 'No one criticizes my boy.' I beamed with pride" (Vance, 2016).

To Danger

Vance describes himself as having left behind aggression as the response to affront. An example he provides, however, suggests the opposite:

> A couple of years ago [note, publication was 2016, when he was 32], I was driving in Cincinnati with Usha, when somebody cut me off. I honked, the guy flipped me off, and when we stopped at a red light (with this guy in front of me), I unbuckled my seat belt and opened the car door. I planned to demand an apology (and fight the guy if necessary), but my common sense prevailed and I shut the door before I got out of the car. Usha was delighted" (Vance, 2016).

Responding to a cut-off and a flip-off by stopping, unbuckling, opening the door to get out, planning to demand an apology and fight if rebuffed is quite far beyond common sense and maintaining control. That Vance would write of this as an example of progress that "delighted" his wife is striking.

For Trump, the path is clear in the response to the 2020 presidential loss, hunkering with a small group of enablers—Giuliani, Clark, Flynn, and the rest; fermenting a narrative of a stolen election; escalation from the demand of, "I just need 11,780 votes" to the threat from a sitting president to the Georgia Secretary of State that he was guilty of, "engaging in criminal acts, baselessly claiming election workers were 'shredding ballots' ... [and alleging] the secretary was covering it up" (ABCNews, 2021).

Going back to his talk of a "homeland" in his Republican convention acceptance speech, Vance makes clear the progression from isolation to othering to danger, from us versus them to, "people will not fight for abstractions, but they will fight for their home," (Bouie, 2024). The progression was manifested in Vance's targeting of Haitian "migrants" in Springfield, Ohio, posting unsubstantiated rumors that, "... my office has received many inquiries from actual residents of Springfield who've said their neighbors' pets or local wildlife were abducted by Haitian migrants. It's possible, of course, that all of these rumors will turn out to be false." However, he extends the targeting with, "Do you know what's confirmed? That a child was murdered by a Haitian migrant who had no right to be here," (apparently referring to a bus accident) (Maher, 2024).

Tailspin

As I wrote in the *Dangerous Case* in 2017, "the more the individual selects those who flatter him and avoid confrontation, and the more those who have affronted and been castigated fall away, the narrower and more homogenous his network becomes, further flattering the individual but eventually becoming a thin precipice," (Fisher, 2017). From General Mattis to Laura Loomer. With this and increasing perceived affronts, and even the risk of prison time, Trump's long and manifestly dangerous behavior—100 police injured defending the Capital on January 6th, several dead—has been widely seen as accelerating.

In his own way, Vance too has shown reactions of anger or disparagement of others in response to stress or challenge. A reporter offered a "softball" question, "You have been criticized as being a little too serious, a little angry sometimes. What makes you smile? What makes you happy?" Vance responded, "Well, I smile at a lot of things including bogus questions from the media, man," ... "as he proceeded to laugh" (Blanchet, 2024).

Different Backgrounds to Shared Current Danger

With their different backgrounds, Trump and Vance each adopted the dangerous combination of isolated grievance that turns almost exclusively to aggression as a tactic. With their statements and, in the actions of Trump on and around January 6th, they have made clear their willingness to extend this pattern into the White House.

As this is written, there is a remarkable example of Trump's and Vance's convergence around danger. During the September 10 presidential debate, Trump took up Vance's accusation of Haitians killing and eating house pets in Springfield, Ohio, still insisting on this after correction by the debate moderator. He and Vance continued with this argument in their appearances over the several days following the debate. In response to continued web traffic promoting the lies, Vance tweeted, "keep the memes coming." Trump continued with a clear threat on September 13 as he, "vowed to conduct a mass deportation from Springfield," (Jordan & Baker, 2024) even though the Haitian people of Springfield are legal immigrants. Far from harmless talk, schools and government buildings have been closed in response to bomb threats (Jordan & Baker, 2024). The rhetoric put targets on Haitians before an audience of 67 million debate watchers as well as those receiving Trump's and Vance's subsequent messaging, continuing to promote what city officials and even the Republican governor of Ohio have confirmed as accusations with no factual basis. From their very different backgrounds, they have each come to assiduously promote the same dangerous myth.

They have also joined to recruit millions of our fellow citizens to celebrate in a perceived isolation and grievance and willingness to attack the "them" who are not "us." The world once again shudders.

Edwin B. Fisher, Ph.D., is a Clinical Psychologist and a Professor in the Department of Health Behavior in the Gillings School of Global Public Health at the University of North Carolina at Chapel Hill. He is a past President of the Society of Behavioral Medicine and editor of Principles and Concepts of Behavioral Medicine: A Global Handbook *(Springer, 2018). In addition to community and peer support in health and health care, asthma, cancer, diabetes, smoking cessation, and weight management, he has written on concepts of psychopathology, including depression and schizophrenia, and on the relationships between mental health and physical disease.*

References

ABCNews. (2021, January 3). Trump demands Georgia secretary of state find "enough votes to hand him win."

Bandura, A., & Walters, R. H. (1959). Adolescent aggression: A study of the influence of child-training practices and family interrelationships. Ronald.

Blanchet, B. (2024, August 12). John Oliver clowns JD Vance for giving "worst possible answer" to a "pretty easy question". *Huffington Post*. Retrieved from https://www.huffpost.com/entry/john-oliver-jd-vance-what-makes-you-smile_n_66b-9b39ae4b00087b34792cb

Bouie, J. (2024, September 14). Shouldn't JD Vance represent all of Ohio?" *The New York Times.* bRetrieved from https://www.nytimes.com/2024/09/14/opinion/jd-vance-haiti-ohio-immigrants.html?smid=nytcore-ios-share&referringSource=articleShare&ngrp=mnp&pvid=283D30B9-5150-4FD5-A70F-63B9E7D8D6A3

Fisher, E. B. (2017). The loneliness of fateful decisions: Social and psychological vulnerability". In B. X. Lee (Ed.), *The dangerous case of Donald Trump: 27 psychi-*

atrists and mental health experts assess a president. Thomas Dunne, St. Martin's Press.

Gaffey, C. (2017, May 25). Trump left Sean Spicer, a devout Catholic, out of meeting with pope at Vatican. *Newsweek.* Retrieved from https://www.newsweek.com/donald-trump-pope-francis-sean-spicer-vatican-615234

Jordan, M., & Baker, P. (2024, September 14). Bomb threats and the FBI: Springfield disrupted by Trump's false migrants claim. *The New York Times.* Retrieved from https://www.nytimes.com/2024/09/13/us/politics/biden-trump-haitian-immigrants-cats-dogs.html?searchResultPosition=1

Lee, B. X. (Ed.). (2017). *The dangerous case of Donald Trump: 27 psychiatrists and mental health experts assess a president.* St. Martin's Press.

Maher, K. (2024, September 10). Vance says false claim he spread against Haitian migrants may not be true but urges followers to keep posting "cat memes". Retrieved from https://www.cnn.com/2024/09/10/politics/jd-vance-haitian-immigrants/index.html

Trump, M. (2020). *Too much and never enough: How my family created the world's most dangerous man.* Simon & Schuster.

Vance, J. D. (2016). *Hillbilly Elegy.* Harper Collins.

Yilek, C. (2024, August 29). JD Vance says Kamala Harris "can go to hell" over Afghanistan withdrawal. *CBS News.* Retrieved from https://www.cbsnews.com/news/jd-vance-kamala-harris-can-go-to-hell-afghanistan-arlington-cemetery/

GODS AND GODDESSES IN THE 2024 PRESIDENTIAL ELECTION

Thomas Singer, M.D.

Our Leaders Live Inside Us

In 2016, I added a post-script to a chapter entitled "Donald Trump and the American Collective Psyche" that I had contributed to *The Dangerous Case of Donald Trump*. I wrote:

> One of the most disturbing thoughts to me about the looming Trump presidency is that he is going to take up residency not just in the White House, but in the psyches of each and every one of us for the next several years. We are going to have to live with him rattling around inside us, all of us at the mercy of his impulsive and bullying whims, shooting from the hip at whatever gets under his skin in the moment with uninformed, but cleverly calculated inflammatory shots. The way a President lives inside each of us can feel like a very personal and intimate affair. Those who identify with Trump and love the way he needles the "elites" may relish having him live inside all of us as a reliable tormentor of those they hate, fear, and envy. Trump is very good at brutally toying with his enemies which include women, professionals, the media, the educated classes, and minorities— to mention just a few.

> What most frightens me about Trump is his masterful skill at invading and groping the national psyche. His capacity to dwell in and stink up our collective inner space is like the proverbial houseguests who overstay their welcome. And many of us never invited Trump into our psychic houses in the first place. That is perhaps why the image that has stayed with me the most from the national disgrace that was our election process in 2016 is that of the woman who came

forward to tell her alleged story of being sexually harassed by Trump. Some years ago, she was given an upgrade to first class on a plane and found herself sitting next to "The Donald". In no time at all, he was literally groping her all over—breasts and below. She describes the physicality of the assault by him as like being entangled by the tentacles of an octopus from whom she was barely able to free herself and retreat to economy class. It now feels as though we have all been groped by the tentacles of Trump's octopus-like psyche that has invaded our psyches for the last year, and that threatens to tighten its squeeze on our collective psyche for at least the next four years. To be as vulgar as Trump himself, Trump has grabbed the American psyche by the "pussy".

Isolation and Despair

At the time I wrote that (2016), I didn't know how long Trump's occupancy in our inner psychic houses would last—but it has been far too long. In the agonizing weeks before July 21, 2024, when Joe Biden stepped down from running for President, Trump's stranglehold on our individual and collective psyches seemed to be tightening into a death grip as his ascendancy to a second term was beginning to seem inevitable. Biden and the Democrats were moribund. Trump was leading in all significant polls, survived an assassination attempt as a hero blessed by God, and was soaring at the Republican convention, basking in the adulation of being a resurrected Christian savior. I found myself becoming increasingly despairing and feeling more and more isolated as I began to think about what a Trump second term might be like: rounding up 10 million immigrants for deportation; gutting many government agencies such as the Environmental Protection Agency, The Department of Health and Human Services, the Department of Education; severely curtailing women's rights to make choices about their own bodies and enthroning himself as an untouchable ruler of a Christian nation. It felt certain that our most cherished values of fairness, equality, decency, and justice would vanish at the hands of an ignorant, but clever autocrat whose nastiness, vulgarity, brutality, selfishness, and truly diabolical nature knows no bounds. (I could well be diagnosed by one of the few Trumpian psychiatrists as suffering from Trump Derangement Syndrome.)

At one point prior to Biden's stepping down, I wrote to a friend:

I feel sick about Biden. I feel sick about Trump. I feel sick about my country. The sickness is a mixture of deep weariness and physical nausea. I fear that something

in me has gone dead with all this--it seems like a huge melodrama in which nothing is what it seems, a great big play signifying nothing. I am wondering if whatever faith and passion I have placed in our 'democracy' may be deserting me now. I am wondering if it is time for me to let it all go. It all feels like a giant charade, even though I know so many of the issues are real and important. Trump is going to come out as a world peace candidate and it is going to get even more surreal as these two old goats, old white men as many of us might say, fuck around with all of us. Perhaps it is just the dystopian mood that has taken hold of me, but I am wondering if it is time to retreat from the affairs of the world. I am thinking that I am going to have to adopt a new attitude for what remains of my life and find a way to disengage from the suffering of the world. It is hard not to take personally the way Trump lives inside me. We may have to live with this pseudo patriot and reality TV star playing the role of hero for an America that has lost its moorings....
Signed,
Old man Tom

My good friend responded:

Tom, re-consider. You're beginning to sound like Macbeth!
'Tomorrow, and tomorrow, and tomorrow,
Creeps in this petty pace from day to day,
To the last syllable of recorded time;
And all our yesterdays have lighted fools
The way to dusty death. Out, out, brief candle!
Life's but a walking shadow, a poor player,
That struts and frets his hour upon the stage,
And then is heard no more. It is a tale
Told by an idiot, full of sound and fury,
Signifying nothing.'
-Macbeth

Yeats' speaker had a different take:
'An aged man is but a paltry thing,
A tattered coat upon a stick, unless

Soul clap its hands and sing, and louder sing
For every tatter in its mortal dress.'
Keep singing, Tom!

The Difference Between Individual Isolation/Despair and Collective Belonging/Hope: The Birth of Gods and Goddesses

Kamala Harris is the one whose soul began to clap its hands and sing for all of us. She has lifted my soul and my spirits as I feel myself joining so many others who were also in isolating despair. And here is the two-part song I am now singing along with Kamala and the millions of others who have found the kindling of hope just as it looked as if everything was going to hell.

1. The first song, a kind of collective "blues", is about the isolating effects of dystopia.
2. The second song is a more celebratory spiritual about the birth of goddesses and gods in Ancient Greece and the modern world. (I have edited a series of books on Ancient Greece/Modern Psyche.)

Why do I spend so much time writing about my own desperation before Biden stepped down and Kamala came to re-energize so many of us? Because I learned something in those despairing moments about the isolating effects of a dystopian mood (something that Black people, women, and so many other oppressed minorities have known about for a long, long time). When we get caught in a dystopian mood, we begin to retreat inside ourselves and feel more and more isolated. We begin to believe that we carry the weight of the world on our shoulders alone, and that it is too much to bear. When Biden stepped down, my feeling of isolation and carrying the weight of the world vanished (Hopefully Biden will come to feel this way, too?) I became more emotionally aware that I was not isolated in the way I thought I was, that literally millions may have felt isolated in exactly the same way I did—alone, hopeless, and carrying an unimaginable weight on our individual shoulders. The effect of Kamala's "taking the torch" was almost instantaneous, as millions emerged from the shadows of their growing dystopian nightmare to embrace hope for a future that may not be terrible. The spontaneous emergence of so many people from the paralysis and disengagement that goes along with feeling alone and isolated was miraculous.

Quite surprisingly, another thought accompanied this reawakening of hope. I wondered if those who have joined Trump's cult may not have, at least somewhere deep down in the core of their beings, also felt isolated in whatever burden they carried alone until Trump came along and provided a target for their frustrated rage and offered hope of a new world. For a moment, I actually found genuine empathy for those who flocked to MAGA world. Trump must have succeeded in speaking to their isolated despair and brought renewed hope to them by messianically seducing them into joining together with a community of fellow believers. In that sense, both Trump and Harris promise a kind of redemption to their true believers that brings the isolated, despairing individual into a reawakened feeling of energized community.

This leads to my second "song", my final leap in this chain of associated thoughts in response to the collective emotional roller coaster of the last several weeks. Jane Harrison, a legendary Greek mythologist, was among the first in the early days of the 20th century who uncovered a layer of the early ancient Greek psyche that was matriarchal rather than patriarchal. Before Zeus and the other gods of Olympus were born and installed on Mt. Olympus, there was a powerful level of the early Greek psyche that placed its faith in the Mother Goddess. In addition to exploring the matriarchal foundations of early Greek culture, what made Harrison's work so interesting is that she followed the lead of the founder of sociology, Emile Durkheim, and made the revolutionary statement that our gods and goddesses are born out of the personification of collective emotion. What does this mean? It means that when groups of people get together and share potent emotions around particularly meaningful events—such as the agricultural miracle for the ancients of new life getting born in the Spring or the modern miracle of Trump surviving an assassination attempt—they tend to personify this event into a god or goddess. They give the annual rebirth of Spring a name, such as Persephone, the daughter of Demeter, who arises from the grips of Hades, the god of the underground. The celebration of the renewal of the earth in Spring is greeted with deep emotion and this collective emotion takes on the identity of a god or goddess. And what does this have to do with Kamala Harris or Donald Trump? It is not a stretch of the imagination to say that we witnessed the birth of a god and goddess within a week.

First Donald Trump, who has always behaved and thought of himself as a divinity, was reborn in the minds of those who believe in him when he survived an assassination attempt. In the collective emotion and imagination of his followers, he became a mixture of Christ as reborn savior and hero warrior patriot in the mode of the Iwo Jima marines, as if rising from the dead to proclaim, "Fight! Fight! Fight!" Trump finally won his "red badge of courage" which had eluded him in the Vietnam war because of "bone spurs" in his feet. But, perhaps even more miraculously, when another old Titan, Joe Biden, realized that his time was up and "passed the torch" to Kamala Harris, she was instantaneously reborn as a warrior goddess, ready to take on Trump who would simultaneously be making his claim to be the resurrected god.

Listen to Kamala Harris speaking as if she might be an incarnation of the Indian goddess Durga who, through her power and strength, will protect her people by slicing through to what is direct and essential about a matter:

> I prosecuted predators who abused women, fraudsters who ripped off consumers, cheaters who broke the rules for their own gain. So, hear me when I say I know Donald Trump's type.

And later when Trump challenged the legitimacy of Kamala's racial identity, Kamala again cut through to the core of her adversary when she said, "The same old show of divisiveness and disrespect."

I am not just speaking metaphorically when I talk about collective emotion fueling god-like projections. Obviously, Trump and Harris are not gods; they are human beings. But the collective emotion pouring onto them makes them seem much larger than life, as if they have drunk the elixir of immortality. According to Jane Harrison, this is how the earliest Greek gods and goddesses found their way into being in the human imagination. As we are witnessing right now, the energy released in these projections of collective emotion is astounding because it has all the numinous power of a religious experience dressed up in political garb. We shouldn't fool ourselves. These are the emotions that fuel religious passions and contribute to the creation of gods and goddesses in the minds of human beings. This election will not be determined so much by specific policies (not to underestimate the emotions about abortion on both sides of the debate), but more on the emotions swirling around these two quite different humans who can easily seem like gods/goddesses. This notion of collective emotion fueling the genesis of gods and goddesses is certainly not the only idea about where divinity originates, but in this situation, it seems particularly applicable. We now have a would-be Christian national savior pitted against a multicultural Black Indian Goddess Warrior, and it promises to be a fully engaged battle led by two very different kinds of people with quite different notions of politics, of government, and of what spirit will prevail in our land.

Thomas Singer, M.D., is a psychiatrist and Jungian psychoanalyst practicing in San Francisco. His interests include studying the relationship between myth, politics, and psyche in The Vision Thing *and* Ancient Greece, Modern Psyche *series. He is the editor of a seven-volume series of books exploring cultural complexes that includes* Cultural Complexes and the Soul of America *and the just-published* Cultural Complexes and Europe's Many Souls: Jungian Perspectives on Brexit and the War in Ukraine. *He is currently President of National Archive for Research in Archetypal Symbolism (ARAS), an archive of symbolic imagery that has created* The Book of Symbols.

TIME AND THE TRUTHS OF TRUMP'S TRAUMATIC IMPACT

BETTY TENG, L.C.S.W.

In 2017, for the first edition of *The Dangerous Case of Donald Trump*, I wrote a chapter titled "Time, Trauma, Truth, Trump." In it, I spoke from my perspective as a trauma therapist, asked to comment on the intense negative impact Donald Trump's 2016 election had on my patient population, the majority of whom are survivors of sexual assault and intimate partner violence. For them, the presidential election of Trump, a known sexual perpetrator and brazen "pussy-grabbing" misogynist, meant that in voting for him, millions of Americans expressed that they did not recognize, care about—or worse, even endorsed the kind of dehumanizing harms that caused the traumas my patients struggled daily to overcome.

And yet, what I also noted—and was puzzled about—was that it was not only survivors of sexual assault who felt shock, fear, anger, and confusion following Trump's 2016 election, but many others as well. My colleagues and I observed the responses in our patients and ourselves as echoing symptoms incurred by traumatic events such as terrorist attacks and natural disasters. "Whatever one's political leanings, one could not equate Trump's win with an actual physical attack or a natural catastrophe," I wrote, "Or could one?" (Teng, 2017). At the time, I observed that with Trump as president, we were in "uncharted territory":

How a New York City real estate magnate and reality television celebrity who had no previous legal, legislative, government, or foreign policy experience could become president of the United States is a circumstance many still find difficult to comprehend. If we agree that the skills of a U.S. president are as crucial as that of a heart surgeon—whose professional judgment and expertise can mean life or death for his or her patients—then it is terrifying to see that the American body politic has, in Donald Trump, a cardiac surgeon who has never set foot inside an operating room. He is a doctor who has no knowledge of, and arguably no interest in, the inner workings of the American government's heart. It therefore makes sense that his lack of qualifications and his insensitivity to the complexities and impact of his role would inspire great anxiety, if not even panic, in those of us whose lives depend on his care—regardless of political affiliation or trauma history (Teng, 2017).

The act of looking back and reflecting on a crucial moment years later offers many things—distance, perspective, understanding. Every four years in the U.S., our presidential elections function as transitional processes that call on us to account for how we, as a nation, might want to cross over into the next interval of time together.

One of the particularly unique aspects of this 2024 presidential election season is that it is not only causing us to look back over the last four years to 2020's decision between Donald Trump and Joe Biden, but even further, to Trump's anomalous 2016 election to the presidency in the first place. This could be due to the fact that Trump is again the Republican nominee, and he is in another tight race against an historic and experienced female opponent, Vice President Kamala Harris. It could also be because, in spite of being voted out of office in 2020, he is back seeking re-election. Underlying all these echoing circumstances is another baffling, if not absurd mystery.

It relates to the question I mulled over seven years ago: if Trump's 2016 election to president was so shocking that it inspired trauma symptoms in so many of us, how is it that he is so close to being elected again?

To help clarify this mystery, I invite us to imagine a modern-day Rip van Winkle—a person who has been asleep for the last eight years, who knows nothing of what has happened in the world. If Mr. van Winkle just woke up and we told him the barest of facts—that Donald Trump was U.S. president between 2016-2020, then lost to Joe Biden in 2020, and now, in 2024, he is again in a close race for re-election, Rip might reasonably conclude that Trump must have done a pretty good job governing during his term. We would then have to inform Mr. Van Winkle that on the contrary, the situation was quite the opposite—that in fact, Donald Trump was a disastrous president. We'd tell him that among a myriad of misdeeds, Trump mishandled a global pandemic, reversed international progress on climate change, and faced impeachment not once but twice, the second time for inciting insurrection on January 6, 2021, when he encouraged thousands of armed white nationalists to block Congressional ratification of Joe Biden's election. This would likely cause Rip to drop his jaw and exclaim, "That makes no sense—what is going on here?"

Indeed, what, actually, *is* going on?

While it may seem insane that we face the stunningly illogical possibility of again electing, as president, a candidate who has already shown himself to be harmful in the role, it is in fact crucial that we face the root of this circumstance. If we, as a democracy, are close to re-electing a deceitful, power-hungry man who has been explicit, in word and deed, about his authoritarian opposition to democratic process, then as much as we like to consider ourselves a nation of immigrants and a haven for the world's most vulnerable, we are also a country of racist, misogynistic xenophobes, who are suspicious, if not hostile, to difference. This reality points to essential truths of our historical traumas, which we as a society have turned away from. Our avoidance has given Donald Trump and his supporters the opportunity to exploit its resulting cycles of shame and blame, polarizing us to a, point where our democracy teeters on the brink of breakdown.

Looking back upon 2016 with the perspective time affords, we might now see that something was way off, that somehow things had gone very wrong. Indeed, for millions of Americans to vote for Trump meant that they either did not take his candidacy seriously or, more troublingly, they actually wanted as president someone brazen enough to act upon their like-minded, in-group grievances and rage. In retrospect, that so many voted destructively rather than constructively, meant that our democracy was in far more peril than we thought.

We might now be able to read more clearly, in our trauma responses to Trump's election, our distress at recognizing how starkly divided we Americans actually are. That some people suffered somatic PTSD-like symptoms in the weeks afterward, signaled how primally Donald Trump's messages were of exclusion and annihilatory threat. Trump's subsequent actions throughout his presidency—from his anti-Muslim travel ban to his insistence on funding for an anti-immigrant wall in Texas; from his refusal to censure violent white nationalists marching in Charlottesville, VA, to his inciting anti-Asian hate by calling the Covid-19 virus the "China-flu"; from his rescinding federal rights for trans individuals to his taking credit for doing away with Roe v. Wade—bore out his threats and validated fears that Trump would misuse his power as president to attack and harm any group he and his supporters deemed as lesser, different, or "other."

85

We can consider this recent history and still feel amazed. We might again echo Rip van Winkle and ask, "Just what is going on here?" even adding, "this is not who we, as Americans, are." But then again—isn't it? Time grants us the distance to see what the past eight years have taught: that indeed, this is also who we, as Americans are. This dark truth is the painful and scary reality Trump and Trumpism call upon us to face. The fact that we, as a nation, are again close to granting Trump the immense power of POTUS, this time knowing full well he will use it to enact further abuses against his opponents and individuals from non-mainstream groups, confirms this.

While such realizations are so alarming that they threaten to shut down thinking, what is crucial to note is that these sentiments are far from new, and that Trump provokes tensions that have existed for centuries. In fact, the depth of our distress and the persistence of Trump's popularity point to the historical wounds and anxieties underlying both.

Indeed, there is much real cause for Americans to feel legitimately fearful and aggrieved. Climate change and a proliferation of ever-more deadly natural disasters caution that our current way of life is unsustainable. Healthcare and prescription drugs are becoming increasingly unaffordable, deepening our sense of physical and economic insecurity. The actual purchasing power of middle-class wages has declined over the last two decades, while the wealthiest among us take an ever-larger share of the country's economic output. Advances in technology, most recently with the expansion of AI, are rapidly changing how we learn and gather information.

Yet, instead of directly addressing these real concerns, Trump instead focuses on blaming undocumented immigrants, women, Blacks, Asians, Muslims—people of any minority identity—capturing the energy of our fears and channeling them into divisive scapegoating. The effectiveness of Trump's tactics reveals the power of the deeper and darker anxieties, which stem from our unresolved historical traumas.

In 2021, in response to a question about how we Americans heal from our collective trauma due to the pandemic, seminal trauma treatment scholar (and *Dangerous Case* co-author) Judith Herman said, surprisingly, "I would argue we are still dealing with the legacy of our Civil War" (Herman, 2023). Psychologist Pauline Boss, who coined the term "ambiguous loss," agrees, "We are a nation founded upon unresolved grief," (Boss, 2023). Both support assertions by psychoanalyst Jessica Benjamin on the conditions for true repair:

We have to have a notion that these things that we're talking about that are so problematic in our history that we, collectively as Americans—both those who did participate in slavery and genocide through their ancestry and those who did not—have to take responsibility for reparation, for making amends, for making sure this doesn't happen again... The less acknowledgment, the less there is what we consider to be repair (Benjamin, 2023).

All point out a truth of American trauma and subsequently, of ourselves: as a society, we Americans have not fully accounted for our traumatic legacy of enslaving and dehumanizing African-Americans for hundreds of years, or for displacing and exterminating Native Americans and appropriating their homeland. As Benjamin points out, this lack of acknowledgement blocks full repair, causing deep collective conflicts to repeat. Moreover, as a protection against guilt, such avoidance incubates anxieties of illegitimacy, which subsequently create defensiveness around privilege.

Yet because the admission of wrongdoing to the monumental crimes of American slavery and the expulsion of Native Americans is too overwhelming, avoidance of a full reckoning has persisted throughout American history. As a result, a vicious cycle continues to churn, as manifested by the entrenched impasses, polarizations and conflicts which characterize U.S. politics today. Of particular note, with respect to Trump's popularity is the legitimating power of grievance and victimhood. Because the very foundation of the United States rests upon these unresolved and unrepaired perpetrations—having grievances and identifying as a victim can allay, if not absolve, in some Americans, the deep, dissociated guilt and sense of illegitimacy we may hold for enjoying benefits historically derived at the cost of subjugating others. As a master of grievance, Donald Trump is expert at claiming the legitimacy of victimhood and of absolution for himself and his followers. This is particularly important for Trumpists now, at a time when assumptions about the primacy of whiteness—and the demographics to support them—are waning.

We can thus recognize in this vicious cycle of dissociated guilt, blame, shame, and fear the psychological and emotional dynamics driving the fierce impasses that have become more commonplace in American politics since 2016. Like the increasingly powerful hurricanes that mark the mounting dangers of climate change, these breakdowns in U.S. government have intensified, manifesting in the form of congressional gridlock, federal shutdowns, and most destructively, in the January 6th insurrectionist attack on the U.S. Capitol. They, too, signal that such tensions are overheating our political ecosystem to a point of no return. As *Boston Globe* columnist Michael Cohen presciently observed in 2020:

> Americans are scared of the wrong things … They're scared about Russia, China and North Korea, when in fact, they should be scared about the fact that … they're politically polarized ... political polarization [is] a big threat to America (Cohen, 2023).

Indeed, Trump has exploited our fears and amplified our grievances, making the divisions between us far worse. He derives and maintains his influence by fomenting "us / them" splits, inspiring cult-like, in-group loyalty among his followers. This not only blocks our ability to communicate and collaborate with each other, it breeds a sense of mistrust and fear in those different from ourselves, creating a catastrophic social cancer that can erode the health of any democracy, never mind one as large and diverse as that of the United States.

Such severe conflicts and divisions indicate that American democracy is in fact very ill, and a second Trump presidency will likely put it on its deathbed. To cite Kamala Harris, we must learn from the recent past and in this election season, take Trump, "an unserious man" (Harris, 2024), far more seriously than ever before. The lessons of 2016 and 2020-21 teach us that, in spite of Trump's chaotic and catastrophic single term as president, and in spite of his shameless disrespect for the rule of law, some of us can still obscure the obvious reality of his dangerous unfitness and consider him a viable candidate for the most powerful leadership position in the world.

While it is crucial to place all our energies into the crucial task of electing Kamala Harris as our 47th President, we must still contend with the root causes of what has brought our democracy so close to the brink of destruction. If we are to stop the harmful creep of authoritarianism in American politics, it is imperative that we find a way out of the vicious cycles that create the conflicts and impasses that threaten our democracy. While noxious and even baffling, these repetitions—which include Trump's viability as a presidential candidate for the third election season in a row—nevertheless clue us into crucial truths about ourselves and the unresolved traumas we must face. For Trump, by channeling his followers' frustrations into potent outlets of white-identified anger, indignation, shame and blame, paradoxically draws our attention to their resolution. To truly heal our ailing democracy, we as a society must undertake the difficult but essential process of making reparations for our original American sins—the historical traumas of slavery and Native American genocide. This is what time and the truth of Trump's traumatic impact teaches us.

Betty P. Teng, M.F.A., L.C.S.W., is a psychoanalyst and trauma therapist who works with survivors of sexual assault, domestic violence, and childhood molestation. A co-author of The Dangerous Case of Donald Trump, *Ms. Teng is a contributing essayist to Adam Phillips'* The Cure for Psychoanalysis *and, with Dr. Tom Singer and Jonathan Kopp, Co-Editor of* Mind of State: Conversations on the Psychological Conflicts Stirring U.S. Politics and Society, *a book based on the psycho-political podcast, "Mind of State." As a faculty member at the Manhattan Institute of Psychoanalysis, Ms. Teng sees couples and adults in private practice.*

References

Benjamin, J. (2023). Acknowledging harm & repairing the world. In Teng, B., Kopp, J., and Singer, T., eds., *Mind of state: Conversations on the psychological and political conflicts stirring U.S. politics & society*. Asheville, NC: Chiron Publications.

Boss, P. (2023). Ambiguous loss & the 2020 pandemic. In Teng, B., Kopp, J., and Singer, T., eds., *Mind of state: Conversations on the psychological and political conflicts stirring U.S. politics & society*. Asheville, NC: Chiron Publications.

Cohen, M. (2023). Analyzing the 2020 election. In Teng, B., Kopp, J., and Singer, T., eds., *Mind of state: Conversations on the psychological and political conflicts stirring U.S. politics & society*. Asheville, NC: Chiron Publications.

Harris, K. (2024). Democratic National Convention presidential nomination speech [speech transcript]. New York Times. https://www.nytimes.com/2024/08/23/us/politics/kamala-harris-speech-transcript.html

Herman, J. (2023). Our collective trauma. In Teng, B., Kopp, J., and Singer, T., eds., *Mind of state: Conversations on the psychological and political conflicts stirring U.S. politics & society*. Asheville, NC: Chiron Publications.

Teng, B. (2017). Time, trauma, truth, Trump: How a narcissistic world leader freezes healing among the traumatized and promotes crisis. In Lee, B. X., ed., *The Dangerous Case of Donald Trump: 27 Psychiatrists and Mental Health Experts Assess a President.* New York, NY: St. Martin's Press.

BEING A CITIZEN THERAPIST IN THE LARGER WORLD

William J. Doherty, Ph.D.

(This is a lightly edited excerpt from the original essay,
"New Opportunities for Therapy in the Age of Trump.")

Donald Trump has done me the favor of helping me to better see the connection between psychotherapy and democracy. In fact, there is a close connection between the personal-agency focus of psychotherapy and the work of democracy understood not just as an electoral system but as collective agency for building a shared life in community (we-the-responsible-people). In our offices, we promote the kind of personal agency that's necessary for a self-governing, democratic people—a people whose worlds are public as well as private. In other words, we are growing citizens of democracies. And therapy needs the larger system of democracy in order to thrive; I've trained therapists who went home to dictatorial systems that greatly inhibited what these therapists could encourage their clients to say and do in their social world.

But to really fulfill the potential of our professional role in a democracy, we have to be active outside our offices. I feel passionately that we're healers with something important to offer our neighbors and communities. Here's a short definition of the concept of the citizen therapist: A citizen therapist works with people in the office and the community on coping productively with public stress and becoming active agents of their personal and civic lives. Citizen-therapist work is not separate from the traditional practice of psychological and interpersonal healing—it's integrated with it.

As an example of citizen therapist work in today's toxic public environment, I've been doing depolarization workshops with "Red" and "Blue" Americans. One stands out in particular: 13 hours over a December weekend in rural Ohio with 11 Hillary supporters and 10 Trump supporters. The goal was to learn if people could better understand their differences (beyond stereotypes) to see if there were common values, and to share, if possible, something hopeful with their community and the larger world. For me, it was like couples therapy with 21 people—intense, painful, illuminating, and ultimately gratifying. After a second, equally successful weekend in southern Ohio, a new action-for-depolarization group has formed of "Red" and "Blue" citizens—a chapter of a national organization called Braver Angels (https://braverangels.org). I've also developed a series of different kinds of workshops and trainings, offered through Braver Angels, that therapists can learn to conduct in their local communities.

The era since Trump calls therapists beyond the personal/public split, a blind spot that has kept us from engaging in comprehensive care for people who bring to us their whole selves, private and public, intimate and civic. It is an invitation to expand and enrich the work we do for our clients and communities.

William J. Doherty, Ph.D., is an emeritus professor of family social science at the University of Minnesota. In May, 2016, he authored "the Citizen Therapist Manifesto Against Trumpism," which was signed by over 3,800 therapists. He is a cofounder of Braver Angels, an organization devoted to depolarizing America at the grass roots level, which is now up to over 4,000 workshops. He helped pioneer the area of medical family therapy, and in 2017 received the American Family Therapy Association Lifetime Achievement Award. His latest book is Becoming a Citizen Therapist, *coauthored with Tai Mendenhall, published in 2024 by the American Psychological Association. Website: https://dohertyfoundation.org/*

THE PROSPECT BEFORE US

Hattie Myers, Ph.D.

Our country is in a dangerous state; democracy hangs on a thread, and trust and truth are in short supply. We are all struggling. Toward this end, I will offer a few things I have learned as a psychoanalyst and as editor-in-chief of an interdisciplinary magazine that engages others, paves a direction, and offers hope.

During the days following the 2016 U.S. election, a cloud hung over New York City. The streets were quiet. On sidewalks, strangers made eye contact with each other. Some shook their heads and shrugged their shoulders. It reminded many of us of what it was like right after September 11.

That week my institute called a community meeting because it was clear that many of us needed to be together. I recall reading them a few sentences by Jean-Paul Sartre who, in writing of the German occupation in Paris said, "The often atrocious circumstances of our struggle made it possible for us to live out that unbearable, heart-rending situation known as the human condition in a candid unvarnished way." At the meeting analysts did speak candidly about heart-rending concerns related to their patients, children, potential war, and the future of our country. Those analysts who had lived through World War II experienced Donald Trump's election as a harbinger of the end of our democracy. The rest of us didn't yet. We were just stunned. None of us, except those older colleagues who had come from Europe, could imagine then how much worse it would get.

It was a comfort to be in the company of others and hear their thoughts and concerns. By way of continuing this connection, a few of us decided to create a participatory newsletter called *ROOM: A Sketchbook for Analytic Action*. But there was another reason to do this. That same week, a colleague from Minnesota was told that her institute would not publish a psychoanalytic essay she wrote because they deemed it too political.

Like our colleague in Minnesota, many mental health professionals, and most prominently Dr. Bandy Lee, would soon come to be dismissed by the media and professional organizations for using their expertise to assess, understand, and even predict some of our country's basic needs. In addition, there was a long-held belief in our field that culture and politics were not relevant in the formation of our psychological realities, and should hold no place in our psychoanalytic theories about human suffering. Against this quiet backdrop of societal trauma and censorship, we moved our analytic work out of the consulting room and published our first issue.

ROOM believes that strengthening connections within communities by sharing meaning where we find it *is* analytic action and that it is part of our professional responsibility to open our office doors to the street. Our first issue carried essays such as "Some Reflections on the New Normal" and "A View of the Election from the Outposts of Old Age" as well as a stirring poem written for the occasion of Trump's inauguration entitled "The Theft Outright." We were shocked that our small newsletter resonated so quickly with so many and now, eight years later, has been read in 160 countries.

ROOM's unique analytic foundations and editorial process remain true to our understanding as psychoanalysts of how change happens. We have come to appreciate the power of an openly participatory democratic process in creating what the Tate Museum has termed a new "Social-Turn Art": a category of art that focuses on constructive social change and is "collaborative, participatory, and involves people as the medium or material of the work." Each of the 24 issues we have published stands, as the first one does, as a moment in time: a witness and reminder of what we have traversed together.

So what have we understood about how to live through instability; how to best fight authoritarianism; and how to foster new forms of collectivity?

I began this essay by describing how, after the 2016 US election, strangers met each other's eyes on the streets of New York, and a community meeting was held. In times of perceived crisis, there is an impulse to draw close. But there is a darker side to this impulse. Drawing close to others when we are destabilized also serves to explain the hold conspiracy theorists and populist leaders have, as well as the hold entrenched party affiliations have had in our divided nation. In stark contrast, connecting with communities that encourage diversity and divergent views strengthens our sense of self and increases our understanding of others. It is the cornerstone of participatory democracy. It is the only authentic safeguard we have against authoritarianism in this country.

My work within *ROOM*'s growing worldwide community has also taught me the importance of supporting those individuals most impacted by authoritarianism. We have published writing from young women in Afghanistan whose futures were snatched from them in a single night, from a psychiatrist in Moscow whose efforts to emigrate with her children have been dashed again and again, from a whistle-blowing journalist in Turkey, and those in Ukraine, Palestine, Syria, and Israel, who write through drone and missile attacks. Fighting authoritarianism means holding space that honors individual resilience and gives wing to imprisoned voices. There have been times their courage has given all of us at *ROOM* strength to continue. I do not take the privilege of being able to publish in this country lightly.

I would like to conclude by sharing a recent extraordinary example of community-building with you. This year, *ROOM* introduced two senior analysts to each other, one from Palestine and the other from Israel. They decided to engage in letters, which we published, and recently we filmed them in conversation in the video, *Speaking of Home: An Intimate Exchange on Israel-Palestine.* Their work poignantly illustrates how there are aspects of ourselves that are *only* available for us to know through conversation with another person. Healing the world requires finding new ways to connect to the parts of ourselves and others that we have been blind to. Joining together in spaces of diversity and divergence creates the possibility for a new collective. Our country depends on it.

Hattie Myers, Ph.D., is a Training and Supervising Analyst at the Institute for Psychoanalytic Training and Research (IPTAR) and Founder and Editor-in-Chief of ROOM: A Sketchbook for Analytic Action. *She has served on the faculty at IPTAR, the Institute for Contemporary Psychotherapy, the National Institute for the Psychotherapies, and New York University School of Social Work, and is past Co-Director of the IPTAR Clinical Center. She co-edited the books,* Terrorism and the Psychoanalytic Space *and* Warmed by the Fires: The Collected Papers of Allan Frosch. *Most recently, she has authored chapters and presented papers on the relationship between Dante and Freud.*

GIVEN HIS LIABILITIES, WHY WOULD WE ALLOW DONALD TRUMP TO LEAD US?

Richard Wood, Ph.D.

Malignant narcissism (Fromm, 1964) can be conceived as a variant of the human condition which arises from profound, severe early trauma. In Trump's case, that trauma appeared to take the form of what Shengold and Shaw have referred to as soul murder, a term meant to capture the devastation that the destruction of one person's subjectivity by another creates. They conceived of soul murder as the most devastating psychic trauma one can endure, as I do. Soul murder was occasioned by a brutal father whose intransigent ascriptions of toughness, ruthlessness, and contempt created a terrible dilemma for his son: either surrender and let the monster who was invading him define him, replicating the actualities that father possessed, or he could resist, attempting in the process to create his own identity— but as a consequence face psychic annihilation perhaps much like his "weaker" brother did. It may well be that Donald's natural proclivities for combativeness and assertion better equipped him for identification with father than brother Freddie's, inadvertently exposing Donald to the devastating loss of self that soul murder imposes.

Becoming tough and ruthless like father and as relentlessly acquisitive was a Faustian bargain indeed. In order to be safe, Trump had to be willing to sacrifice his connection with others and his very humanity. To ensure he could never be invaded again and defined by someone else, he had to hold himself apart from meaningful engagement with other people, maintaining a tough guy posture, much like his father had, that denied need, dependence, and recognition of his own flawed humanity, all the realities that are

96

an inherent part of the human condition and that render life meaningful and sustaining. Instead, he embraced the grandiosity that his father had imparted. He became a world and a law unto himself. Never again would he have to accommodate others' voices or feel violated by them; never again would he have to accommodate another personality, allowing himself to be shaped by another person or touched and moved by them. He could become a world unto himself. And in that world, there would only be room for one voice and one self: his own. Others would have to accommodate themselves to his vision, his prerogatives, and his agendas. Never would he have to make room for them. Locking himself up in his own "house" in this way meant that he would have to deny himself bonds of affection, empathy, and love. Love implicated weakness. Love would connote invasion, diminishment, and obligation to others and shared interdependence, none of which he could embrace without compromising the grandiosity and invulnerability so important to him and so necessary to protect him and hold him together. His relationships, of necessity, had to become utterly transactional, zero-sum games in which he always dominated and he was always the perceived winner. If others shared his rapacities, a relationship could persist; once that actuality ceased to exist, there was no accrual of value built upon depth of regard for the other. Others could be valued, after a fashion, however, if they showed themselves willing to twin themselves with him, ready to swallow holus bolus the varied "truths," beliefs, and doctrines he presented, however transitory they might be.

In the malignant narcissist's world, everyone is a potential enemy. Everyone is experienced by Trump as being as rapacious and avaricious as he is. There is no real safety to be afforded except by confirmation of one's ability to overpower others. Rapacity and avariciousness grow out of the fear of violation that his original traumatizing experiences etched indelibly into his soul, a kind of identification with the original aggressor— you do unto to others before they can do unto you. It also derives, very poignantly, from the devastating starvation Trump must endure. Without love, compassion, and gratifying interdependencies, Trump cannot fill himself. He must relegate himself, instead, to pursuit of alternative forms of sustenance— fame, money, power, and acts of cruelty and domination— to nurture the self. These are forms of sustenance that can never nourish and satisfy, setting the stage for rage and for devastating envy of others' decency and of love that he can never have for himself.

To protect the self, someone who is malignantly narcissistic like Trump must needs adopt a war footing, ready to engage in relentless and merciless combat with others he experiences as encroaching upon his prerogatives and his exclusivity of identity. Perpetual combat, particularly of a sort that is characterized by a need to crush other personalities, ensures that one's world is soon replete with real enemies. It also means that one's inner world feels evermore dangerous as well, littered, as it is, with both the shattered remains of his victims and the specter of ever-present warfare.

In a 2016 article, psychologist Dan P. McAdams referenced a quote attributed to an interview Trump did with People Magazine in 1981 "Man is the most vicious of all animals, and life is a series of battles ending in victory or defeat." Trump is telling us that he lives in a very Darwinian, visceral world in which dominance and subjugation provide the only avenue to survival. In order to traverse such a world and even flourish in it, one must, of necessity, be able to act with alacrity, with ruthlessness, and without hesitation. Empathy must be neutered. Unyielding self-interest must predominate. Neutered empathy and perceived self-interest become unselfconsciously enacted habits of being that come to be almost casually directed towards one's fellow human beings.

Consider but a few of many telling examples. Trump's family separation policy directed towards prospective immigrants attempting to cross the Mexican-US border was initially conceived as a way to leverage Democrats and some resistant Republicans into acceptance of the administration's tough immigration policies. As a result, 2300 children were separated from their families; only after profound outcry was his policy reversed, but, even so, several hundred children still remain cut off from their parents. There was no apology or expression of regret from Trump or his administration, either to the general public or to the families that had been injured.

On June 1, 2020, a crowd of peaceful protesters outside St. John's Episcopal Church was dispersed by police and National Guard who used smoke canisters, rubber bullets, batons, and shields so that Trump and some administration officials could proceed to the church steps for a photo op in which Trump posed holding a Bible. Again, there was no recognizant expression of regret or remorse about the people who had been injured or terrorized as a result, and no recognition that excessive force had been used.

The Trump administration relentlessly attacked Obama's Affordable Care Act, seemingly because it represented an Obama rather than a Trump proposal. As a result, millions of people who previously enjoyed healthcare, including women and children, were excluded from same. The alternative health care act that Trump and Paul Ryan enthusiastically propounded, in turn, would have, astonishingly, denied healthcare coverage for 23 million Americans. Absent was an expression of concern about the jeopardy people subjected to these policies would have to endure.

Mismanagement of the Covid 19 crisis in April 2020 resulted in the US having the highest official death toll of any country in the world; during this extended crisis, Trump promulgated dangerous, "quack" cures for the nation to rely on and appointed advisors, like Michael Caputo, to disrupt accurate dissemination of information about the crisis that Anthony Fauci was charged with conveying to the public. Trump offered no apology and expressed no regret about the harm that his policies had caused or the potential damage that his intemperate health advice had occasioned.

And then there were the deliberate acts of cruelty and tenacious vendettas that Trump seemed to relish. Personal vendettas against people like the *New Yorker* writer Gail Collins (a dog with a pig's face) and/or broader ones directed towards larger groups of people ("shit hole" countries or admonitions to George Floyd demonstrators that if they breached the White House fence they would be "greeted with the most vicious dogs and most ominous weapons I've ever seen"). Acts of cruelty simulate aliveness and engagement that would otherwise be realized through depth of connection, which is inaccessible to the malignant narcissist.

Turning away other people's voices, creativity, and expertise, particularly in the context of unyielding personal aggrandizement, places someone like Trump in the position of making evermore extravagant errors of judgment. He imagines that because he says things or does things or sees things in a particular way, they must be true simply because he is special and so his thoughts and actions must be. He fractures rationality because it suits some transactional end for him to do so. He may also do so, however, simply because he "feels" something in a given moment— again, the premise being that that which emanates from him must be precious. At times his aggrandizement of his ideas and his productions expresses contempt for those who would believe him; more ominously, it also reflects the ease with which he can get lost in his own ideas and distortions of truth, experiencing them as realities that ought to be honored (transitory delusional states). All of these factors further contribute to the likelihood, as he becomes progressively trapped in his own grandiosity and his solipsism, that the errors of judgment he makes will become increasingly intemperate and dangerous— errors of judgment in a leader of the most powerful country in the world that have the potential to cause great harm, particularly in a personality bereft of love, empathy, and compassion. Even more concerning, as his errors of judgment accumulate and become more transparent, his efforts to protect his grandiosity become evermore desperate. His grandiosity, after all, is the glue that holds him together. While we see that Trump's sense of grandiosity is remarkably resilient in the face of the many challenges that have been turned against it, it is important to keep in mind that it can fail him and that such failure will likely represent a catastrophic psychological experience, much like the annihilatory anxiety he must have endured during his growing up years as his father made perpetual efforts to crush him. In such a context— if, for example, the idealization of his core followers is replaced with jeering, derision, and laughter— Trump is likely to experience such an annihilatory event. Malignant narcissistic leader personalities conflate personal identity with national identity. Suicidal despair in such people connotes extreme risk for anyone whom they might harm. In a man who holds the nuclear triggers of one of the world's largest nuclear arsenals in his hand, this is indeed a sobering prospect.

So why do malignant narcissistic leaders attract so many devout followers? Composing a credible answer will surely reflect, as it must, as much about the realities and vulnerabilities that we all carry inside us as it does about the malignant narcissist himself.

A leader like Trump engages so many of us because he speaks to our alienation— underlying sources of injury, fear, uncertainty, inadequacy, and inequity. Real calamities, such as war, profound economic reversals, threats to cultural integrity, acts of widespread prejudice and hatred, widescale threats to health, etc., etc., all lay the groundwork for a sense of alienation that can be exploited. In the absence of such imposing threat, a malignant narcissistic leader may create threats that don't exist (but that feel credible), or exaggerate ones that are genuinely present. It would be fair to say that Trump has done both. Malignant narcissistic leaders rely upon fear to draw their followers towards them. In acknowledging the fear that they elaborate or exacerbate, personalities like Trump establish a sense of empathic attunement with those that they seek to seduce. He is seen to understand the untoward realities that people feel characterize their lives that no one else has been willing to address. Make no mistake: his empathy is an empty vessel defined only by his desire to acquire more of the goods he values— fame, money, power, etc.

Trump further consolidates his purchase with his intended followers by speaking with great authority. He is the only one, he tells those he would entrance, who is equipped to solve the alarming problems that he has been perceptive and empathic enough to identify. An air of certitude and authority is very powerful. The Milgram experiments (1963), which have been replicated in a variety of forms, show us that even bright, well-educated people are willing to inflict lethal levels of harm on others simply upon receiving instruction to do so from an authoritative other. Adorno (1950) made us aware that certain cultural practices that typify a given culture may contribute to culture-wide receptivity to an authoritarian voice. Lifton (2017) draws our attention, in turn, to the concept of malignant normality. Malignant normality refers to the idea that we can become inured to acts of inhumanity and indecency because they are so widespread in a given culture, they have been normalized by it. Hannah Arendt's concept of the banality of evil (1963) asked us to consider that many of the people who perpetrate evil at the direction of others are possessed of rather quotidian personalities themselves. Her formulation, however, also foreshadows, to my mind, the Lifton concept. We don't see, think about, or feel the implications of that which is so commonplace to us. We are drawn instead by our membership in our home culture to accept cultural practices as a means of affirming our belonging to our group and our identification with it. In my first two books, *A Study of Malignant Narcissism: Personal and Professional Insights* and *Psychoanalytic Reflections on Vladimir Putin: The Cost of Malignant Leadership,* I emphasize the importance of group belonging and identity as an immensely important driver of human behavior as, indeed, have many other writers. Dispossessed people that Trump addresses have now been given a righteous cause to pursue: make America great again, a harkening back to imaginary better times that Trump promises to restore. Joined by unity of purpose and a nostalgic re-invocation of an idealized past, they can restore meaning, pride, and sense of community, by any measure a very powerful inducement to draw them into MAGA. The vague promises and abstractions which Trump provides allows his listeners to project whatever they might wish into that vision of better life.

Very fundamentally, Trump is inviting his followers to partake in the grandiosity and implied power of his dominance and his authority. They, too, can feel bigger than they have been, more expansive, more influential, if only they would twin themselves with his priorities. Once they have done so, they must be careful never to step outside the bounds of discretion and judgment that he prescribes for them, especially as he expands his power. Their voices must align themselves with his. Authoritarian leaders— which I believe Trump is— consolidate their authority through the invocation of fear. To disagree is to face censure, punishment, or even the threat of physical reprisal. Followers have already been asked to turn their wrath towards those whom he would target. He has asked the attendees at his rallies to direct physical force against hecklers; his invocation at the January 6 insurrectionists to "fight like hell" led to widespread physical violence, six deaths, and 138 injuries to police officers, some of them severe.

There is another powerful reason people are drawn to movements like MAGA.

It frees them from having to accommodate accountability for their own actions. They no longer have to mediate their own impulses, deciding what is moral and what is not. The leader makes those choices for them, deciding when it is appropriate for them to unleash the malignant parts of themselves that we all carry inside and when it is not.

As malignant narcissistic personalities consolidate their control of a given society, progressively devastating voice and democratic process, which we can see Trump has more or less continuously attempted to do in his first term, fear and repression become ever more prominent characteristics of day-by-day life. Like the malignant narcissist, everyone begins to feel alone, no one feels safe, and everyone struggles with the fear that the leader's wandering hatreds can direct themselves towards them. The malignant narcissist typically pulls this structure together by creating enemies, both internal and external, towards whom people can direct their growing rage and fear. As they do so, their internal worlds increasingly begin to replicate his, marked by growing and ever-expanding hatreds and prejudices. Disturbingly, in mid-August 2019, the Brookings Institute shared FBI data that confirmed a spike in hate crimes in counties that voted predominantly for Trump.

Truth; factuality; science; thoughtful, nuanced response; and appreciation of complexity all endure depreciation under malignant narcissistic leadership. In their place, decision-making driven by affects like fear, hatred, and bigotry assume ascendancy. Thinking becomes more binary, marked by simplistic distinctions between good and bad, friend versus foe, good versus evil, facilitating prejudicial acts and decision-making which serves the malignant narcissist well in his pursuit of perpetual warfare.

It is hopeful that we know so much more about malignant narcissistic leaders and the leader-follower relationship. We are now in a far better position to forewarn ourselves and to identify dangerousness in the people who would lead us. We must recognize the need to bring cultures of caring forward, so the people don't feel left behind and neglected. We must also more deliberately encourage people to think critically, educating them to do so and giving them license to stand apart, speaking their own version of truth. Constructing an environment that is more respecting of individuality and voice and of individual difference would certainly make it easier for these things to happen. And, lastly, as imperfect as it is and as aspirational as it is, we must be far more mindful than we have been about protecting democratic process. We must continuously remind ourselves that democracy, as Ian Hughes has suggested (2018), probably evolved as a defense against malignant leadership.

Richard Wood, Ph.D., received his baccalaureate from Cornell and his doctorate from Wayne State University. He served as Staff Psychologist at Mount Sinai Hospital, Associate Professor in the Department of Behavioral Science, University of Toronto Medical School, and in private practice. He was President of the Ontario Psychological Association, a Founding Member of the Canadian Association of Psychologists in Disability Assessment. He was Director of the Thornhill Multidisciplinary Assessment Center. He is author of three books, A Study of Malignant Narcissism: Personal and Professional Insights, Psychoanalytic Reflections on Vladimir Putin: The Cost of Malignant Leadership, and Narcissism, a Contemporary Introduction.

References

Adorno, T. et al (1950). *The Authoritarian Personality.* New York, NY: Harper & Brothers.

Arendt, H. (1963). *Eichmann in Jerusalem: A report on the banality of evil.* New York, N.Y.: Penguin.

Diamond et al. (2022). *Treating Pathological Narcissism with Transference Psychotherapy.* New York and London: The Guilford Press.

Fromm, E. (1964). *The Heart of Man.* New York, N.Y.: Harper & Row.

Hughes, I. (2018). *Disordered Minds: How Dangerous Personalities Are Destroying Democracy.* Winchester, U.K. & Washington, USA: Zero Books.

Kernberg, O. (1984). *Severe Personality Disorders.* New Haven, Conn: Yale University Press.

Kohut, H. (1976). Creativeness, charisma, group psychology: Reflections on the self-analysis of Freud. In P.H. Ornstein (ed.). *The Search for the Self* (volume 2, pp.743-843). New York, N.Y.: International Universities Press.

Lifton, R.J. (2017). Malignant normality. *Dissent,* (64)(2), 166-170.

Malkin, C. (2017). Pathological narcissism and politics: A lethal mix. In B., Lee (Ed.). *The Dangerous Case of Donald Trump.* (2nd ed., pp. 88-103). New York, N.Y.: Thomas Dunne Books.

McAdams, D. P. (2016). The mind of Donald Trump. The Atlantic. June 2016.

Milgran, S. (1963). Behavioral study of obedience. Journal of Abnormal and Social Psychology, 67, 371-378.

Rosenfeld, H. (1971). A clinical approach to the psychoanalytic of the life and death instincts: An investigation into the aggressive aspects of narcissism. *The International Journal of Psychoanalysis,* 52, 169-178.

Shaw, D. (2014). *Traumatic Narcissism.* New York, N.Y. and London, U.K.: Routledge.

Shengold, L. (1989). *Soul Murder: The Effects of Childhood Abuse and Deprivation.* New Haven: Yale University Press.

Wood, R. (2023). *A Study of Malignant Narcissism: Personal and Professional insights.* New York, N.Y. and London, U.K.: Routledge.

Wood, R. (2024). *Psychoanalytic Reflections on Vladimir Putin: The Cost of Malignant Leadership.* New York, N.Y. and London, UK.: Routledge.

THE CULT OF TRUMP

Declaring a Public Health Emergency and Psychoeducation is Our Long-Term Solution

Steven Hassan, Ph.D.

In 1974, when I was 19 years old and a junior at Queens College, I was deceptively recruited into an authoritarian mind-control cult—The Moonies. I was radicalized and told to drop out of college and follow God. My freedom of mind was subverted, and a false Moonie version of me was programmed into believing that Sun Myung Moon was the Messiah, and that democracy was satanic. The real "me" was wholly suppressed. My once progressive ideals were replaced with Moon's extremist right-wing beliefs. I worked 18 to 21 hours a day, 7 days a week. I was a true believer willing to die or kill on command. I was made into a leader and trained to subvert American democracy and install a theocracy in its stead.

Fortunately, after a near-fatal van crash due to sleep deprivation, I was deprogrammed. This did not happen with my willing participation, but my parents had forced it on me while I was convalescing. This experience changed my trajectory, and now I am a licensed mental health professional who has dedicated my career to helping others heal from this kind of experience, through my scholarly research as well as education of the public about cults and undue influence.

What is little known is that the Moonies paid Donald Trump $2.5 million to endorse them, and they constitute a significant propaganda force through the publication they operate, the *Washington Times*. The Moon cult has also been at the center of climate science denial for 50 years. I have seen how the agenda I learned about in the 1970's is coming to fruition in 2024.

Erich Fromm coined the term malignant narcissism when he attempted to describe Adolf Hitler. As a cult expert, I can say this *is* the stereotypical psychological profile of every leader I have studied in a destructive, authoritarian cult. In Chapter Three of *The Cult of Trump* (Hassan, 2019) I compared Trump to death cult leader Jim Jones, my former cult leader, Sun Myung Moon, and sci-fi hypnotist cult leader Ron Hubbard of Scientology. My book has stood the test of time and has been thoroughly validated, even down to my prediction that if Trump lost the 2020 election, we should expect violence.

I wrote about the puppet masters of Donald Trump in Chapter Seven of *The Cult of Trump*. Vladimir Putin was at the top of the list of authoritarians who have been busy using him to advance the agenda to undo the U.S. government and its administrative state functions. What is also clear is that many different authoritarian cults comprise a big chunk of the base for the MAGA movement. I wrote about The Family, The New Apostolic Reformation, Opus Dei, Ayn Rand Libertarians, and others. I learned about The Council for National Policy from Anne Nelson, and realized they installed James Whelan as the founding editor for The *Washington Times* newspaper.

Every Republican President has endorsed the Moonie paper since its inception. George H. W. Bush was director of the CIA when the House subcommittee investigation took place into South Korean CIA activities in the U.S., which included the Moon organization. Bush did everything possible to undermine the investigation, which showed that the Moonies were being used as a front group for extremist right-wing forces using anti-Communism to fight "the enemy."

My doctoral thesis demonstrated the first scientifically validated construct for evaluating authoritarian control. Utilizing my Influence Continuum and BITE Model of Authoritarian Control (Behavior, Information, Thought, and Emotion control) provides a framework for updating the law regarding undue influence. At its foundation is the existing law for trafficking, which names Fraud, Force, or Coercion to exert influence over an individual. The BITE Model gives much-needed granular detail to explain these three concepts to judges and juries.

Many people incorrectly assume that destructive cults are all religious, but the BITE Model can be applied to political parties and dictatorships as well. Alarmingly, Trump's most fervent supporters display the profile of destructive cult members. They seem unable to understand that Donald Trump is a pathological liar, but their cognitive dissonance makes them believe he is an agent of God. He is not trustworthy. They deny experts and science. These so-called patriots want to tear down the world leadership status of the USA, demonstrating the power of fourth-generation psychological warfare used on them.

Many reject vaccination against preventable diseases. Donald Trump has them disbelieve any critical media, saying it is "fake news." Their own doubts are suppressed. They think in black-and-white terms, such as us versus them and good versus evil. They are unable to utilize critical thinking skills. Finally, they lash out emotionally and exhibit denial when confronted with facts such as that Trump is a sexual abuser, a 34-time convicted felon, and does not believe in the rule of law. Their emotions of fear and rage are spurred on by propagandist information warfare.

Donald Trump thus can control their thoughts and emotions. He can drive them to action— even to acts of terrorism, such as the violent insurrection attempt of January 6th, 2021. When I was in the Moon cult, I was encouraged to participate in multiple hunger strikes and demonstrations, at significant risk to my own mental and bodily health. I understand how the mind control tools that Trump employs can cause individuals to act out of character, driven by intense zeal and fury. Just because these individuals act out in harmful ways does not mean they are a lost cause. With patience, understanding, and education, I believe they can be freed from this malicious undue influence controlling their thoughts, feelings, and actions.

To bridge the divide in our country, we must develop a wide-scale program to educate everyone about cult mind control. While I dislike the term "deprogram," it is the word the public understands about helping people "start thinking for themselves again." Remember that their true selves are buried under all the conspiracy and paranoia. Media pundits often depict Donald Trump's MAGA followers as permanently brainwashed and unreachable. This is false! I have experienced it firsthand and have helped countless other cult survivors reemerge from undue influence and regain control of their lives. Rational arguments using facts to persuade people to change their minds do not work. Asking respectful questions using active listening works. We must remember that these individuals are our friends, family, and neighbors, and approach them rationally and respectfully. We must build rapport with individuals suffering from cult mind control and illustrate to them that we are worthy of their trust. We need to ask them important questions such as:

- How did you come to believe what you now believe?
- If you decide to change your political alignment, can you do this safely?
- What criteria would you feel are valid for exiting the MAGA group?

By remaining respectful and asking questions, we can encourage them to think critically about the issues and idols that now dominate their lives. We can begin to understand what led them down the dark Trump conspiracy rabbit hole and dismantle their destructive mindset to hopefully create an opening for their authentic self to shine through.

We can inoculate the public against their mind-control techniques by creating countermeasures to stop the spread of disinformation and encouraging media literacy through Public Service Announcements (PSAs) and public education. With openness, education, and understanding, we can convert Donald Trump's most ardent supporters and depolarize the nation, hopefully restoring truth, justice, and hope to this great country again.

Steven Hassan, Ph.D., is a mental health professional, forensics expert, and Fielding Fellow who has been helping people leave destructive cults since 1976. He founded and directs the Freedom of Mind Resource Center, Inc. He is the author of Combating Cult Mind Control, Freedom of Mind, *and* The Cult of Trump. *He has been featured in major media outlets such as the Associated Press, the Wall Street Journal, CNN, ABC, NBC, and the New York Times. He has developed "the BITE Model," the world's first scientifically validated construct for evaluating authoritarian control and hosts the podcast "The Influence Continuum."*

EVANGELICALS DO NOT SEE TRUMP FOR WHO HE REALLY IS

—And It is Causing Great Harm
to Our Country and the Cause of Christ

CHRIS THURMAN, PH.D.

(A lightly edited version of this article was originally published in Salon on March 29, 2024, and is reprinted here with permission.)

I have been largely apolitical throughout my life. All of that changed when Donald Trump came down the escalator in Trump Tower to announce his candidacy for President of the United States in 2015. Over the months that followed his announcement, I became increasingly alarmed by the political rise of Trump and the evangelical support he garnered. It was clear to me at the time that Trump was intellectually, psychologically, and morally unfit for office, and that it was delusional for anyone, especially evangelicals, to think otherwise.

My alarm only grew as increasing numbers of evangelicals threw their support behind Trump with his selection of Mike Pence, a devout Christian, as his running mate. It was at that time I began to write opinion pieces criticizing Trump and challenging evangelicals to stop buying into his self-glorifying lies. With very few exceptions, my op-eds fell on deaf ears.

Fast forward to today, and the unfitness of Trump to occupy the Oval Office is only worsening, as is the delusional view many evangelicals have of him. MAGA evangelicals, like lambs led to the slaughter, continue to believe the things that come out of Trump's mouth, something deeply concerning, given that he is widely seen as a pathological liar.

From my perspective, evangelical support of Trump in 2024 falls into the category of, "Fool me once, shame on you. Fool me twice, shame on me." Shame on Trump for malevolently conning evangelicals into supporting him in 2016. Shame on evangelicals for being conned back into supporting him in 2024, given his catastrophically bad presidency and noticeable unfitness for office. There are none so blind as those who will not see, and Trump-supporting evangelicals are among the most blind Christians to ever engage in politics.

Before going any further, I want to define *delusional* as I'm using it in this article. A person being delusional is "characterized by or holding false beliefs or judgments about external reality that are held despite incontrovertible evidence to the contrary." It is my contention that many MAGA evangelicals are delusional about Trump in that they continue to see him in an extremely positive light, even though who he is and how he acts would suggest seeing him in an extremely negative one.

Along these lines, Trump-supporting evangelicals are especially good at cherry-picking verses from the Bible to justify their support of Trump, but they seem to have a strong aversion to dealing with passages of Scripture that clearly warn against doing so. I believe there are two primary biblical passages that argue against supporting Trump for president. In focusing on these passages, I have two questions I would like evangelicals who support Trump to answer.

How do you support someone for president who unrepentantly practices the things God hates?

One of the most important passages in the Bible for understanding Trump, one that MAGA evangelicals often ignore, is Proverbs 6:16-19. It says:

There are six things the Lord hates, seven that are detestable to him: haughty eyes, a lying tongue, hands that shed innocent blood, a heart that devises wicked schemes, feet that are quick to rush into evil, a false witness who pours out lies, and a person who stirs up conflict in the community.

From my perspective, this is a word-for-word description of how Trump operates.

1.   Trump has haughty eyes in that he proudly believes he never does anything wrong. Trump once said he had never asked God for forgiveness because he hadn't done anything bad enough to warrant it.

2. Trump has a lying tongue. During his presidency alone, he told over 30,000 lies, and the frequency of his lying has only increased since he left office.

3. Trump's gross mishandling of the COVID crisis qualifies as the shedding of innocent blood. Tens of thousands of people died unnecessarily from COVID, all because Trump didn't want the numbers to make him look bad.

4 & 5. Trump has a heart that devises wicked schemes (scam schools and charities); and feet that are quick to rush into evil (affairs, tax evasion, sexual assault, defaming others, inciting an insurrection).

6. Trump bears false witness against others in that he frequently attacks people's character, especially the character of those he feels the most threatened by, in an effort to distract from how little character he possesses.

7. Finally, Trump stirs up conflict wherever he goes, disunifying our country every step of the way.

Evangelicals, how do you support someone like this for president?

How do you support someone for president whom God says to ignore?

A second passage for understanding Trump that many of his evangelical supporters refuse to acknowledge is 2 Timothy 3:1-5. It is, from my perspective as a psychologist, a description of a malignant narcissist:

There will be terrible times in the last days. People will become lovers of themselves, lovers of money, boastful, proud, abusive, disobedient to their parents, ungrateful, unholy, without love, unforgiving, slanderous, without self-control, brutal, not lovers of the good, treacherous, rash, conceited, lovers of pleasure rather than lovers of God—having a form of godliness but denying its power. *Have nothing to do with such people* (italics mine).

I would argue again that this is a word-for-word description of Trump.

Trump exhibits malignant narcissism in that everything is about him and how great he thinks he is. Trump is a lover of money in that he has lived his adult life greedily pursuing wealth, and behaving as if he can never have enough. He is beyond boastful, talking ad nauseum about how he knows more than all the experts in their respective fields. Trump is abusive, especially when it comes to the verbal and emotional abuse he inflicts on those around him. He is unforgiving and has already warned us that if elected president for a second term, he is going to be a dictator on day one and go on a revenge tour against his enemies, the likes of which our country has never seen. Trump lacks self-control in many areas of life including food, sex, golf, and reigning in his tongue. He clearly isn't a "lover of the good." To the contrary, he seems to have a strong penchant for loving evil and evil dictators in what guides his actions. Finally, Trump portrays himself as a godly man when there is no substance behind it. Trump recently said he was proud to be a Christian, something no right-minded Christian would say, and he has been out hawking Bibles lately while portraying himself as someone who loves the Word of God. All of these actions reflect Trump trying to appear to be someone he's not—a God-fearing, Bible-loving man who models his life on the life of Jesus Christ.

Evangelicals, how do you support someone like this for president?

No matter what the cost, Christians must stand up for truth.

It is not inherently delusional to hold conservative *or* liberal values. Both sides of the political aisle have core values that are admirable and worth fighting for. What turns holding these values into something problematic is when a person or a group of people take them to radical extremes and weaponize them for personal gain and glory, while not caring about the damage they cause the country in the process. Trump and his MAGA evangelical supporters are such people, and, consequently, I believe it is both foolish and delusional to support him holding the highest office in the land.

I have great admiration for Nathaniel Manderson's opinion piece in Salon magazine, "My calling as a Christian minister: Stand up against evangelical hypocrisy." I admire any Christian who is willing to risk being attacked and vilified when he or she feels other Christians are in error and need to be called out for it.

I identify with many of the things Manderson said about the price one pays for speaking out against Trump, and the hypocrisy and blindness of evangelicals who support him. Personally, it has been painful for me to lose friendships and some degree of professional respect over my criticisms of Trump. But, as is the case with Manderson and many others who have had the courage to oppose Trump and his followers, I'm far better off not having certain people as friends, or the regard of certain professional colleagues, if they are unwilling to respectfully and rationally engage in *truth-based* debate about whether or not Trump is fit to lead this country.

Within the body of Christ, there appears to be little willingness to reason anymore, and unbridled emotions seem to be running the show. We are deeply divided as to whether or not supporting Trump is wise or foolish, biblical or unbiblical. But this is part and parcel of how Trump operates—sow discord and division among groups of people, even Christian groups he claims to identify with, and ride that division all the way to the White House for personal glory and not the glory of God.

I think our country is strong enough to withstand another Trump presidency. But, to be honest, I do not want to find out. It is a risk we cannot afford to take. I respectfully ask Christians who support Trump to reconsider. The stakes are incredibly high in every election but are especially high in this one. If you are conservative like me, please consider voting for someone else in November. Please vote for someone who, though imperfect like all of us, *genuinely* cares about truth, doing good, the sanctity of human life, compassion for the downtrodden, and unifying our country, not someone like Trump who gives the appearance of doing so for self-serving gain.

Chris Thurman, Ph.D., is a psychologist, former professor, and author of numerous books, including The Lies We Believe *and* Emotionally Healthy Christianity. *In 2020, he organized and published* The Spiritual Danger of Donald Trump: 30 Evangelical Christians on Justice, Truth, and Moral Integrity, *for which he invited Dr. Bandy X. Lee to write the prologue. He draws upon his Christian faith to offer help and hope to people. He has a B.A. in psychology from the University of Texas at Austin, an M.S. in counseling from East Texas State University, and a Ph.D. in counseling psychology from the University of Texas at Austin.*

Reference

Manderson, N. (2024, March 17). My calling as a Christian minister: Stand up against evangelical hypocrisy. *Salon*. Retrieved from https://www.salon.com/2024/03/17/my-calling-as-a-christian-minister-stand-up-against-evangelical-hypocrisy/

HOW TRUMP ATTACKS OUR CAPACITY FOR COMPASSION

Lorne Ladner, Ph.D.

Donald Trump's well-documented mental instability is characterized both by a lack of empathy, normally associated with pathological narcissism, and a lack of compassion, normally associated with sociopathy and sadism.

Sadism is the polar opposite of compassion—delighting in causing others' suffering and humiliation. Adam Serwer, journalist at the *Atlantic*, wrote a popular essay entitled "Cruelty is the Point" in 2018, followed by a book of the same title in 2021. He explores the history of cruelty in American politics with Trumpism as its current, extreme expression. Our concern should not only be about Trump's own sadism and how extremely dangerous it is when combined with great power, but also how the Trump movement directly undermines and attacks our own capacities for empathy and compassion. It is easiest to begin developing compassion when we feel interpersonally safe, relatively calm, and connected with others as we take time to empathize with them. A rhetoric of suspicion, divisiveness, cruelty, and rage is a direct attack on our capacity for compassion. Trump exploits his followers' emotional vulnerabilities in ways that decrease their capacity for compassion. This "anti-compassion" effort includes campaigns of misinformation to create an atmosphere of threat; overt expressions of intense destructive emotions such as contempt, sadism, and hate, which evoke similar emotions in those who listen to him regularly; and systematic efforts to undermine the sense of interconnectedness, pitting native born against immigrant, conservative against liberal, White against Black, men against women. Those efforts on his part along with additional, overt attempts to provoke fear, anger, agitation and disgust, also affect the capacity for compassion of those of us who see his dangerousness and oppose him politically.

In Abraham Lincoln's first inaugural address on the eve of the Civil War, he pleaded with his fellow Americans, "We are not enemies, but friends. We must not be enemies. Though passion may have strained it must not break our bonds of affection." Compassion grows from affection and recognition of our common humanity. Since the Trump Contagion (Lee, 2024) undermines those qualities not only in those who vote for him but in all of us to some extent, cultivating affection and compassion for each other must be an essential part of a long-term strategy to healing the mass mental disturbance that afflicts our nation.

Since the Trump Contagion spreads not only by way of misinformation but also by the creation of an emotionally toxic environment, in which destructive emotions like rage, hate, fear and paranoia predominate, inoculation against it requires not only calling out lies and inaccurate information but also creating an emotional environment restorative of positive emotions such as love, compassion, and joy. I learned about the power of this approach from Ribur Rinpoche, a Tibetan Buddhist monk whom I met when he came to teach at a Buddhist center in California. Early in his life, when the Chinese Communist army invaded his country, he was captured and imprisoned for being a prominent Buddhist lama. During Mao's Cultural Revolution, soldiers who were caught up in the contagion of misinformation and rage of that time tortured him for years in prison and dragged him through the streets, in attempts at public humiliation. Rinpoche, who became a dear mentor and friend, said that although his body suffered a great deal during those years, his inner experience was, "nothing but pure joy." As a psychologist working in the suburbs of Washington, DC, I had regularly seen people with remarkably comfortable outer circumstances who are extremely depressed and even suicidal. In hearing of Ribur Rinpoche's experience, I became fascinated by how a person could experience precisely the opposite of that: being in the worst possible outer situation while internally experiencing joy.

When Rinpoche was in his 80's, he developed cancer. I was with him over the course of a year as he went to oncology appointments, had medical procedures, and received chemotherapy. I watched carefully as he exhibited remarkably heartfelt peace and joy in those circumstances. One day, I asked him if this resulted from a sort of enlightenment, and he playfully scowled in disagreement. I then thought about my years of knowing him, and I asked if it really derived from his deep practice of loving compassion. He smiled very broadly at that. He noted that it is not very effective if you wait to take up training in compassion until things are terribly difficult and painful, as then it will be quite difficult to give rise to such feelings. However, if you train regularly in cultivating compassion when you feel relatively safe and calm, then when things get difficult, compassion will provide a refuge. He noted that if you have trained well in compassion beforehand, then compassion only grows stronger when faced with your own or others' suffering.

The nature of compassion is wishing to relieve the suffering of the world, so actually feeling some of that suffering directly is like adding fuel to the fire of compassion. It also became clear that Rinpoche's compassion practice was what had inoculated him against the madness of the Cultural Revolution. Even when faced in very direct, personal ways with the hatred, paranoia, and rage of Mao's Cultural Revolution, he felt compassion for his fellow prisoners of conscience and also for the soldiers and Red Guard members who were torturing him and attempting a cultural genocide against his people. Hence, he never fell victim to paranoia, othering, terror, hate, or despair himself. After the Cultural Revolution was over, Rinpoche worked with fellow Tibetans and with Communist officials in helping to restore the most precious sacred arts of his culture.

One point that Ribur Rinpoche emphasized to me, which psychological research has also shown to be true, is that anyone can cultivate compassion. Research also shows that doing so benefits yourself as well as those around you. When I was in medical settings with Rinpoche, numerous medical professionals approached me, sometimes with tears in their eyes, asking how someone could radiate the loving peace he did. The same thing even happened at Dulles International Airport with the workers there. My own experience was that often simply having a quiet cup of tea with him felt emotionally similar to being at a huge, outdoor concert with 20,000 people feeling love as they listened to a favorite, uplifting song.

Researchers have shown the role that mirror neurons play as people have resonant effects with the emotional experiences of those around us. We are all experientially familiar with how being around someone who is utterly enraged can change the feeling in a room. And since Donald Trump has entered presidential politics, we have also all seen how one man's overwhelming experiences of contempt, anger, paranoia, and hate can affect millions of people when it is shared regularly on television and the Internet. Emotional contagion does not only work with toxic emotions; it also is effective with tonic ones. Kamala Harris and Tim Walz have been making an effort to work with that effect in emphasizing joy as part of their presidential campaign. If we wished to counter the Trump movement, then our shared strategy must include decreasing exposure to destructive emotions while increasing private and public expressions of emotions such as loving-kindness, hope, joy, gratitude, and compassion.

Mindfulness is a good starting point for cultivating compassion, because it decreases stress and opens our state to becoming more aware of direct experiences. Direct experience is important in the context of regular exposure to lies and conspiracy theories. The practice of mindfulness begins with focusing attention on the breath and other present-moment sensations, and also seeing our thoughts and feelings for what they are: impermanent things that change with each moment. By practicing mindfulness, we can let go, free ourselves of ruminations on things such as misinformation that others produced to control our minds, and ground ourselves in what we perceive for ourselves at that given moment.

Once you are mindfully present, compassion can be cultivated in a variety of ways. A common element is the recognition that you and others are interconnected, that their well-being and yours are interdependent. Whether you look at the international economy, pandemics, global warming, healthcare systems, gun violence, or efforts towards peace, what is happening could not more clearly illustrate how each of our welfare is more linked to the well-being of others than we usually recognize. A challenge of our time is seeing through how the mass psychosis of psychopathological fascism misrepresents clear illustrations of our utter interconnectedness as reasons to disconnect from and resent each other. For example, global warming clearly illustrates how activity anywhere on the planet affects those everywhere else, and compassionate engagement requires vast cooperation. Instead of promoting such understanding, Trump says that climate change is a "hoax" not worth worrying about, and says, "Great, we have more waterfront property," in reaction to rising sea levels (Pichrtova, 2024). To believe him is quite literally to succumb to delusion.

And if some of our neighbors, family members, and friends have been infected with psychologically toxic input that cause them to see these things precisely as they are not, there is no asylum for such psychosis. Such infections can lead to a sense of alienation and disconnection. The cultivation of compassion requires coming back to a realistic recognition of our interdependence. Martin Luther King Jr. vividly illustrated this when he said, "We are caught in an inescapable network of mutuality, tied in a single garment of destiny. Whatever affects one directly, affects all indirectly," (King, 2024). This is the point Lincoln was making when he called citizens friends with bonds of common affection. It is important to understand that it is not sufficient to simply say, "I have compassion," but rather we must develop an inner experience of compassion, moment after moment. People who experience powerful anger or hatred spend many hours ruminating on their grievances as their brains and bodies habituate to more and more intense agitation. An antidote to that is to repeatedly contemplate how each other person around us is precious, is worthy of affection, and is to be cherished, as our physiology habituates to love. Such love feels warm, joyful, and open-hearted. We then turn that affectionate felicity towards a realistic acknowledgment of how we and others suffer. We also open to awareness of how, although we don't wish to suffer, we too often inadvertently run towards the very causes of sorrow. This sort of awareness tempers our love into something very strong: compassion. Habituating our bodies and minds to such experiential compassion affects us directly and all indirectly, and thus provides hope for healing.

Lorne Ladner, Ph.D., is a clinical psychologist in private practice in Virginia. He wrote The Lost Art of Compassion *and co-authored* Bridges of Compassion *(with Alex Campbell). He wrote a chapter on "Mindfulness" in* Spiritually Oriented Interventions in Counseling & Psychotherapy *and produced a training video on* Mindful Psychotherapy *(with Jon Carlson) for the American Psychological Association Press. He has provided trainings for mental health professionals on compassion and on narcissism as an obstacle to compassion. He has also provided workshops and trainings around the country on mindfulness and the cultivation of positive emotions.*

References

King, M. L. (2024). *Why We Can't Wait*. New York, NY: Random House.

Lee, B. X. (2024). *The psychology of Trump contagion: An existential threat to American democracy and all humankind*. New York, NY: World Mental Health Coalition.

Pichrtova, A. (2024, August 13). Trump says climate change means "more oceanfront property." *Newsweek*. Retrieved from https://www.newsweek.com/trump-climate-change-not-biggest-threat-oceanfront-properties-1938397

PART 3
HARPOCRATES
(GOD OF SILENCE)

THE ETHICS OF APA'S GOLDWATER RULE

JEROME KROLL, M.D., AND CLAIRE POUNCEY, M.D., PH.D.

(This article was originally published in the Journal of the American Academy of Psychiatry and the Law, *44(2), 226-235. It is reprinted here with permission.)*

Section 7.3 of the code of ethics of the American Psychiatric Association (APA) cautions psychiatrists against making public statements about public figures whom they have not formally evaluated. The APA's concern is to safeguard the public perception of psychiatry as a scientific and credible profession. The ethic is that diagnostic terminology and theory should not be used for speculative or ad hominem attacks that promote the interests of the individual physician or for political and ideological causes. However, the Goldwater Rule presents conflicting problems. These include the right to speak one's conscience regarding concerns about the psychological stability of high office holders and competing considerations regarding one's role as a private citizen versus that as a professional figure. Furthermore, the APA's proscription on diagnosis without formal interview can be questioned, since third-party payers, expert witnesses in law cases, and historical psychobiographers make diagnoses without conducting formal interviews. Some third-party assessments are reckless, but do not negate legitimate reasons for providing thoughtful education to the public and voicing psychiatric concerns as acts of conscience. We conclude that the Goldwater Rule was an excessive organizational response to what was

121

clearly an inflammatory and embarrassing moment for American psychiatry.

In 1964 when Barry Goldwater, senior senator from Arizona, was the Republican candidate for the office of President of the United States, *Fact* magazine surveyed psychiatrists' opinions about Goldwater's mental health and published the results.[1] A public outcry ensued, criticizing psychiatrists for publicly proposing pejorative diagnostic and psychodynamic statements about a figure whom they had never formally evaluated. The American Psychiatric Association (APA) condemned the use of psychiatric commentary for political purposes, and nine years later declared unethical psychiatrists' public commentary on public figures who have not been personally examined and had not given consent for disclosure. This dictum, established as Section 7.3 of the APA Code of Ethics,[2] is informally known as the Goldwater Rule.

The facts of the Goldwater case and the controversies surrounding it remain relevant to psychiatrists and the psychiatric profession. A recent article by Cooke *et al.* in the *Journal* uncritically accepts the substance of the Goldwater Rule and sets itself the task of providing a method "that guides psychiatrists in their interactions with the media to help them avoid violating ethics principles or the law."[3] The August 2015 issue of the *American Journal of Psychiatry* carries a three-page commentary discussing and generally supporting the Goldwater Rule.[4] An op-ed article in the New York Times Online of March 7, 2016, by psychiatrist Robert Klitzman of Columbia University provides the background to the Goldwater Rule and supports psychiatrists' compliance with the overall intent of the rule while acknowledging controversies and inconsistencies in its application.[5]

In this article, we look at the scientific and practical concerns related to the nature and rules of evidence and methodology in making diagnoses, and the moral questions related to conflicts for the psychiatrist between codified rules of ethics and various other moral obligations according to private conscience and codes of conduct. We conclude that the Goldwater Rule is not only unnecessary but distracts from the deeper dictates of ethics and professionalism. Our aim is not to endorse self-promotion or grandstanding by psychiatrists, but to question whether the codified Goldwater Rule is too restrictive in cautioning psychiatrists against public commentary and yet too lax to direct individual decision-making.

Psychiatry's Response to Public Embarrassment

Fact magazine, founded by Ralph Ginzburg and Warren Boroson, was a bi-monthly magazine published from January 1964 to August 1967. It ran articles and editorials opposing and attacking conservative politics and policies, among other targets. In July 1964, one week after the Republican Party convention nominated Barry Goldwater as its presidential candidate, Ginzburg sent out questionnaires to 12,356 psychiatrists whose names were on a list purchased from the American Medical Association. The Sept–Oct 1964 issue of *Fact*, published just before the November presidential election, was devoted solely to the Goldwater question. The issue contained a long editorial introduction written by Ginzburg, entitled "Goldwater, the Man and the Menace," and 38 pages of psychiatrists' comments.[1] The cover of the magazine proclaimed: "1189 Psychiatrists Say Goldwater is Psychologically Unfit to be President!" in bold 48-point font.

The survey asked a single question, "Do you believe Barry Goldwater is psychologically fit to serve as President of the United States?" The survey allowed space for additional commentary from each respondent. The actual description of the survey and its methodology and results comprised just three brief paragraphs on one page of the 64-page magazine issue. Of the 12,356 inquiries, *Fact* magazine received 2,417 responses as follows:

1.   Did not know enough about Goldwater: 571
2.   Goldwater psychologically fit: 657
3.   Goldwater not psychologically fit: 1189

There were no percentages or statistical analysis reported, nor any discussion about the validity of a 19.5 percent response rate to a questionnaire, of which only half were negative about Goldwater. Of the commentaries that many psychiatrists included in their responses to Ginzburg's survey, *Fact* published 38 pages in the Goldwater article; some were letters critical of *Fact* for conducting this kind of survey; some contained positive comments about Goldwater's character and mental health; and many were highly critical of Goldwater, with much psychological and psychodynamic speculating, opining, and theorizing. Goldwater was called "paranoid," an "anal character," a "counterfeit figure of a masculine man," and a "dangerous lunatic." He was accused of having a "grandiose manner" and "Godlike self-image," and a "stronger identification to his mother than to his father," and so forth. There was no mention by the editors as to how these comments were selected for inclusion.

Senator Barry Goldwater sued Ralph Ginzburg and *Fact* magazine in federal court for libel. Goldwater alleged that the statements written about him in *Fact* were falsehoods made with actual malice and with knowledge that the statements were false or with reckless disregard of whether they were false or not. A federal jury awarded Goldwater $1 in compensatory damages and $75,000 in punitive damages in 1966.[6] The U.S. Court of Appeals for the Second Circuit upheld the verdict in 1969[7], and the Supreme Court in 1970 denied a petition by Ginzburg and *Fact* magazine for a writ of *certiorari*.[8] Justices Black and Douglas dissented based on First Amendment guarantees giving "each person in this country the unconditional right to print whatever he pleases about public affairs" (Ref. 9, p 1054).

Where the courts were dismissive, the APA was not. In 1973, the APA formalized its condemnation of psychiatrists, publicly commenting on persons whom they never examined and who had not signed a release of information, and included the Goldwater Rule in 1973 as Section 7.3 of the first edition of its Code of Ethics.[2]

Section 7.3 of the Principles of Medical Ethics states in its entirety:

> On occasion psychiatrists are asked for an opinion about an individual who is in the light of public attention or who has disclosed information about himself/herself through public media. In such circumstances, a psychiatrist may share with the public his or her expertise about psychiatric issues in general. However, it is unethical for a psychiatrist to offer a professional opinion unless he or she has conducted an examination and has been granted proper authorization for such a statement.

We read the Goldwater Rule as making three claims: that standard diagnostic practice in the United States requires a personal interview before making a diagnostic formulation; that it is a breach of medical ethics for a psychiatrist to openly discuss the diagnoses and psychodynamics of a person whom the psychiatrist never interviewed and who has not expressly consented to public commentary; and that such behavior of psychiatrists misleads the public regarding the legitimate expertise, function, and methods of modern psychiatry and brings ridicule and shame to the entire psychiatric profession.

This third claim is tacit yet speaks volumes. The psychiatrists who enthusiastically responded to the *Fact* survey with psychodynamic and diagnostic speculation about

Goldwater embarrassed the psychiatric profession. The APA has a legitimate concern that the public not perceive psychiatry as pseudoscientific speculation clothed in diagnostic and psychodynamic terminology.

The APA's Position on the Goldwater Rule

In this section, we present our understanding of the APA's position regarding Section 7.3 of The Principles of Medical Ethics with Annotations Especially Applicable to Psychiatry. We include in this section writings by several prominent psychiatrists who support Section 7.3.

The APA's basic position on diagnostic standards is that a direct psychiatric examination is an integral component of the diagnostic process. Speculating publicly as a psychiatrist about someone whom the psychiatrist has not examined violates professional standards of ethical behavior and undermines the integrity of the standard of psychiatric practices. The APA strongly supports responsible psychiatric education of the public on matters that are of concern to society at large. This includes psychiatrists who speak in public forums and via various media about general matters of diagnosis and treatment, health care risks, relationships of mental illnesses to aberrant public behavior, effects of social disturbances on mental health, and a variety of other topics. It is specifically the types of public statements exemplified by the Goldwater case that the APA condemns. The APA, as an organization, has a responsibility to uphold a positive image of the profession in the public eye. A psychiatrist who disregards the basic procedures of psychiatric diagnoses and treatment, including the proper use of scientific methods in assessing evidence, and acts without discretion and confidentiality, would tarnish the reputation of the APA and the public's trust in psychiatrists.

The public generally assumes that psychiatrists hold a special role in society as experts in human motivation and behavior, which carries a degree of credibility and knowledge above that attributed to ordinary citizens. Because of this presumed expertise, authority is given to the statements of psychiatrists, even when they are acting in the capacity of private citizens. In this regard, the APA, as the professional organization representing the psychiatric profession, asserts that it has the right to establish ethics standards and rules of behavior for its members that may be more stringent or restrictive than the rights allowed by the First Amendment.

Many psychiatrists have articulately defended the reasonableness of the APA position. In 1998, Herbert Sacks, then president of the APA, held that reporting of psychobabble by the media undermines psychiatry as science.[10] The psychobabble of interest at that time involved President Clinton's marital troubles, using such constructs as sexual addiction, narcissism, risk-taking, hyperthermic men, and evolutionary biology, and was reminiscent of the terms used to describe Goldwater in the *Fact* article. Sacks criticized psychiatrists who demonstrated their political partisanship by pushing their agenda in intemperate public displays of metapsychology, psychodynamics, and omniscience.

Richard A. Friedman, professor of psychiatry at Weill Cornell Medical Center and an occasional columnist on psychiatric topics for the *New York Times*, has been a vocal, if selective, defender of the Goldwater Rule. He has strongly opposed psychiatrists' public commentary on American political figures. Friedman, in a column in the *New York Times* in 2011, invoking the Goldwater debacle of 47 years earlier, criticized psychiatrists who offered opinions about Dominique Strauss-Kahn (former head of the International Monetary Fund) and his sexual scandal.[11] In this same article, however, Friedman stated that an exception can be made as "ethically defensible" for psychiatric profiles of foreign political leaders. Friedman proceeds to suggest that Col. Muammar Qaddafi of Libya "has a severe personality disorder called malignant narcissism."

In earlier writing, Friedman abided by the letter as well as the intent of the rule. In response to media disclosures[12,13] of the sexual misdeeds of Eliot Spitzer, the former Governor of New York, in 2008, Friedman wrote that although it would be unethical for a psychiatrist who had never examined Spitzer to claim that he has a narcissistic personality, the psychiatrist, as part of a professional duty to educate the public, could describe a narcissistic personality, while disclaiming that Spitzer is being referenced.[14,15] In the same article,[14] Friedman justified Jerrold Post's testimony, at a 1991 open Congressional hearing, that Saddam Hussein had malignant narcissism. Post had acknowledged that he based his diagnosis on several biographies and interviews with individuals who knew Saddam Hussein. The justification of labeling Hussein and Qaddafi as malignant narcissists in the absence of personal examination was to let Congress and the American public know that these two individuals, as malignant narcissists, have a defect in moral conscience and lack empathy, thereby rendering futile all efforts to appeal to them (and others like them) on human terms. Post viewed this obligation to warn policymakers about Hussein as similar to invoking the *Tarasoff* warning about a mentally ill and dangerous individual. Whatever the political expediency and justification of rendering diagnoses and psychodynamics at a distance, the same limitations of methodology and validity, and the same risk of getting it wrong, were present for Hussein as for Goldwater and Spitzer, except the stakes were higher in getting it wrong about Hussein. Public events often raise questions about the mental health of public figures. Motivations for such public interest reflect, at least in part, our vital stake in the health and behavior of politicians, diplomats, generals, and others whose decisions influence our lives and wellbeing. It makes sense to ask questions of experts in human behavior, and there is a strong case to be made that it is the experts' responsibility to educate the public about human behavior and motivation, just as we expect experts to educate the public on global warming and evolutionary theory. The APA agrees that the profession has an important role in public education about mental health and illness topics. At issue are the questions of what are the proper topics and methods for such education.

Rethinking the APA Position

Our discussion will proceed by challenging the content of the Goldwater Rule. First, we question the APA's position that the standard for psychiatric assessment includes an in-person interview. Second, we consider the propriety of the APA requirement that psychiatrists protect the profession's interests above their own moral commitments.

Finally, we argue that psychiatrists have a positive obligation to speak publicly in many circumstances, and the right to speak out in others.

Claim 1: Standards for Diagnostic Formulations

The Goldwater Rule privileges the personal interview as the standard by which a practitioner may form professional opinions. Clinical impressions, however, can be made to greater or lesser degrees of precision. The most precise is formal diagnosis, which in its most rigorous form requires record review, collateral history, and one or more in-person patient interviews. However, a full history and past records are not always available, and time and distance may impose practical limitations. For clinical purposes, psychiatrists often, appropriately, make do with a single in-person interview, and since the advent of telepsychiatry, interviews may be conducted from afar. There is little theoretical or empirical support for the APA's restrictive claim that only personal examination can lead to valid diagnoses.

For nonclinical purposes, professional diagnostic opinions may be made and confirmed in a number of ways. For example, structured diagnostic interviewing for research purposes may be performed by a clinician, but may also be carried out by having a subject answer questions on a computer. Diagnoses may also be made using filmed interviews of psychiatric research subjects, such as was the case in the classic U.K.–U.S. research studies into transatlantic differences in diagnoses of schizophrenia and bipolar disorder.[17–19] This research provided the basis for a major professional reappraisal by U.S. psychiatrists about the theoretical biases that influence diagnoses of severe psychotic illnesses. In line with this technology, psychiatric board certification required, until recently, candidate psychiatrists to give a formal diagnostic assessment based on a videotaped interview. For administrative purposes, diagnoses are usually made strictly from written records. Insurance companies regularly diagnose mental disorders *post hoc* without in-person interviews, a practice that, if not welcomed by the APA, has not been challenged. The insurance industry routinely uses clinicians who never have examined the patient to determine that person's diagnoses and need for treatment. Vitally important decisions about access to health care are made about patients daily by physicians (not necessarily psychiatrists) as well as nonphysician clinicians (psychologists, pharmacists, and nurses) who have never directly examined the patients and who, by any standards, must be involved in conflicts of interest. The physician, psychologist or nurse who is paid by an insurance company to review medical necessity of hospitalization or outpatient treatment, in full knowledge that at least one of the goals of the review is to keep costs down, is never free from a conflict of interest.

Federal programs as well as private insurers require periodic chart audits and peer reviews to assess diagnostic accuracy and treatment quality in the absence of a personal interview. The APA is silent about these practices.

In psychiatric malpractice cases, psychiatrists proffer opinions as to the diagnoses, dynamics and best treatment protocols without directly examining the patients. This is most obvious in cases involving completed suicides, but also in boundary violation cases, improper pharmacological treatment for a given diagnosis, and other alleged malpractice situations. Chart reviews are accepted as the evidentiary bases for expert opinions.

There is a long academic tradition of psychohistory that requires making psychiatric assessments based on written records and accounts. Freud's Schreber case is the model for formulating clinical opinions about the psychodynamics of a person who has not been personally interviewed.[20] Psychohistory and psychobiography are broadly accepted and respected domains of clinical research in which diagnoses are made and psychodynamics formulated in the absence of personal evaluations. Erik Erikson's biographies of Martin Luther[21] and Mahatma Gandhi[22] and John Mack's biography of T. E. Lawrence[23] are three well-known and respected examples (with the biographies of Gandhi and T. E. Lawrence each winning a Pulitzer Prize), but there are countless more, including Kroll's papers on the medieval mystics Beatrice of Nazareth[24,25] and Henry Suso[26] and the Byzantine Emperor Justin II.[27] Even in biographies of persons who lived centuries ago, the researcher can check and compare numerous sources against each other to increase accuracy and account for authorial bias. The general consensus within the medical and medical history communities (and the Pulitzer Prize committee), at variance to the Goldwater Rule, is that diagnoses based upon records, whether historical or contemporary, written, visual, or auditory, can be as accurate as diagnoses made by direct examination.

Furthermore, personal examinations are notoriously flawed. As a process, a first-person account falls under the category of impression or presentation management, a well-studied field of Social Psychology that examines how individuals try to shape or control the impressions that others form of them. Patient interviews are not fully reliable because of conscious (intentional) and unconscious distortions, which is why thorough diagnosis considers the accounts of other persons and written records. Patients under direct interview or in psychotherapy do not tell the whole story, or the accurate story, or they tell a rationalized and distorted story. In fact, the entire foundation of Freud's theory of the unconscious is that motivations and wellsprings of action are not directly accessible to the person in question, so that patient accounts are necessarily distorted by their psychological defenses. That patients may not respond truthfully to an interview does not entail abandoning first-person interviews as a key component of the diagnosis. First-person testimony is critically important to clinical examination, but it is subject to the unavoidable limitations of all human interactions.

On these grounds we challenge the tenet that diagnostic opinions can be made only on the basis of in-person clinical interviews. Public behaviors can be recorded by examining psychiatrists, by other health professionals, by journalists, and by casual observers. What is unique to psychiatry is the understanding of how those public behaviors may reflect psychopathology.

Claim 2: Conflicts between Professional and Personal Codes of Ethics

The second claim of the Goldwater Rule enjoins psychiatrists to refrain from speaking about public figures unless the examinee has given explicit permission to do so. We consider this requirement in light of other professional and personal moral obligations. We argue that psychiatrists have an obligation to protect the privacy of psychiatric patients, but not the public perceptions of the psychiatric profession. For the Goldwater Rule to dictate how psychiatrists characterize public figures confuses the interests of patients and individual psychiatrists with the interests of the psychiatric profession.[28] Professionalism and professional ethics are related but not identical. Professionalism includes professional etiquette (e.g., dress, hygiene, and manners) as well as the moral code of conduct for psychiatry. Violations of ethics are sanctionable by the profession, but violations of etiquette are not. The Goldwater Rule provides an excellent standard of etiquette, but should not be included in psychiatry's code of ethics.

This second claim is redundant of Section 4 of the APA Code of Medical Ethics. Section 4 establishes that any communication by a psychiatrist about a patient outside of the treatment relationship requires express consent to release protected medical information: "A physician shall respect the rights of patients, colleagues, and other health professionals, and shall safeguard patient confidences and privacy within the constraints of the law."[2] Based on Section 4, it would constitute an ethics breach for the personal psychiatrist of a public figure to speak about his patient without permission.

Section 4 includes a significant caveat regarding legal mandates, such as court orders to disclose private patient information, the privacy of minors, and psychiatrists' legal obligations to protect the public from dangerous persons. Permission for psychiatrists to disclose confidential patient information is recognized in Section 4.3 of the APA Code: "When . . . the risk of danger is deemed to be significant, the psychiatrist may reveal confidential information disclosed by the patient."[2] The duty to protect patient privacy is not absolute, even within the doctor-patient relationship. Without a clearly established doctor-patient relationship, no professional duty is violated, yet the Goldwater Rule applies in these situations.

What is more, Section 7 of the APA Code of Ethics encourages psychiatrists to advise governments and the public [S7.1], and to share "their expertise in the various psychosocial issues that may affect mental health and illness" [S7.2]. It thus reiterates the directive of Section 5 of the APA Code for psychiatrists to participate in public education. Together, these commitments to public education, public health, and social awareness create a mandate for psychiatrists to engage in rather than refrain from commentary when public figures seem to pose a risk to community safety. We see, then, that whereas the Goldwater Rule's first claim (requiring personal examination to form a professional opinion) is not maintained consistently in ordinary practice, the second claim that a psychiatrist may not discuss diagnostic formulations of public figures who have not consented to commentary is redundant of both Section 4 and 5.

Now consider Section 7.2: "Psychiatrists shall always be mindful of their separate roles as dedicated citizens and as experts in psychological medicine".[2]

This reminds psychiatrists that they may not speak about personal commitments in the name of all psychiatry. The code says nothing, however, about what a psychiatrist ought to do when the dictates of those roles compete; there is no widely accepted algorithm for balancing personal against professional obligations. Different social roles may create competing personal and professional imperatives, and choosing to speak out as a concerned citizen, or parent, or member of a religious or other subcommunity may win out over ambiguous professional obligations to remain silent. It is inappropriate for a professional organization to expect, much less require, that professional obligations will trump all other interests.

This may mean that some psychiatrists do embarrass the profession, but doing so is not a breach of ethics. In 2011–2012, the press reported that Newt Gingrich, a serious contender in the Republican presidential primaries, demanded an open marriage from his second wife as the price for not pursuing a divorce. Within 24 hours of this political bomb, which ordinarily would spell disaster to a candidate running on a "family values" platform, Keith Ablow, the in-house psychiatrist for Fox News, asserted in his blog that Gingrich's marital infidelities make him better suited to be President of the United States because it shows he will make a very strong president.[29] Within hours of this statement, Ablow was attacked in the Huffington Post,[30] EqualityMatters blog,[31] and others, but not by the APA. Nor was Dr. Ablow sanctioned for his pseudoscientific commentaries on how parents may create gender identity problems in their children and how transgender individuals do not exist.[32] This sort of psychologizing is what the Goldwater Rule constrains, but the APA did not refer Dr. Ablow to his district branch for investigation of misconduct. The psychiatric community did not need the Goldwater Rule to publicly disapprove of this type of blogging by a psychiatrist, as exemplified by the critical comments made by Jack Drescher,[33] a member of the DSM-5 Workgroup on Sexual and Gender Identity Disorders, and by John Oldham, then President of the APA, as cited in the Gay and Lesbian Alliance Against Defamation (GLAAD) blog.[34] It is important to note that of the dozens of blogs critical of Dr. Ablow, the criticisms were directed toward the individual, and none criticized the psychiatric profession as a whole. It is also important to note that if Dr. Ablow were not a member of the APA, he would not be eligible for professional sanction. This single illustration suggests that, at least in some cases, the Goldwater Rule is both superfluous and impotent.

The Goldwater Rule cannot distinguish between thoughtful and well-researched psychiatric commentary on public figures and the flippant sound bites about celebrities and politicians who make each day's headlines. For the individual moral agent choosing a course of action, the Goldwater Rule provides no direction, except to require that he prioritize the reputation of the profession. The Rule cannot adjudicate which commentaries are responsible and which are spurious, facile, and suspect, so it condemns them all. But every day the public is presented with questions about the psychological health of public figures. If we go further into the past, Woodrow Wilson's stroke; Winston Churchill's bipolar disorder; John Kennedy's Addison's disease; Abraham Lincoln's depression, Marfan's syndrome, or head injury; Hitler's paranoid personality and possible amphetamine addiction; Eisenhower's stroke; and Reagan's dementia all become topics of great interest to those who are concerned about the intersection of health and illness, personality, decision-making, and policies of international import. Miles Shore[35] has provided thoughtful commentary on the success and limitations of this early promise of a collaboration between psychiatry and political science in understanding irrational political behavior.

Psychiatrists are well trained to be public educators, but the Goldwater Rule denies an individual psychiatrist's responsibility to speak up about political leaders' behaviors that strongly suggest psychopathology. Not only does the Rule fail to prevent the embarrassing pseudopsychology promulgated by *Fact* magazine, but it also subdues what could be useful and important public debate. A psychiatrist deciding whether to comment on a public figure in either the popular media or a professional journal must be permitted to balance personal and professional commitments as he sees fit. When these conflict, or when the professional commitments conflict with one another, the individual must adjudicate for himself whether his actions are morally right, and simply hope that no ethics-related charges will be brought. Although the Goldwater Rule sets an appropriately high standard for professional behavior, it is misplaced as an ethic rather than an important guideline for action. Medical school and residency provide most of our education on professional conduct, and learning to think carefully before speaking publicly about public figures could be part of required curricula. To include it as a rule in the APA Principles of Medical Ethics overreaches. We believe that the Goldwater Rule may be considered as one guideline among many, but we do not think it should override other personal and professional obligations. We want to make an even stronger claim. We believe that the Goldwater Rule is itself unethical if it suppresses public discussion of potentially dangerous public figures. There have been serious and well-researched books and blogs by psychiatrists on public figures. A book entitled *Bush on the Couch*, published in 2003 and updated in 2007, was written by the Washington D.C. psychiatrist and psychoanalyst Justin Frank, who is a past president of the District of Columbia chapter of Physicians for Social Responsibility.[36] Frank saw the threat to world peace and security by President George W. Bush acting out his own parental dynamics as so serious that it would be cowardly and immoral for him not to speak up (personal communication, January 13, 2012 and February 26, 2016). Frank has also published an analysis of President Obama (*Obama on the Couch*), in which he offers psychodynamic hypotheses as to President Obama's seeming inability to recognize the implacable nature and uncompromising stance of the opposing political party.[37] The *New York Times* published a letter to the editor by Frank during the 2016 presidential campaign defending the use of "applied psychoanalysis" in assessing political figures.[38]

Jerrold Post, a Washington D.C. psychiatrist who has provided psychological profiles of world leaders for over 20 years for the Central Intelligence Agency, has written several books, articles and media commentaries offering psychological profiling and strategic recommendations for dealing with such figures as Slobadan Milosevic and Radovan Karadzik,[39] and on Yasir Arafat, Osama bin Laden, Saddam Hussein, Kim Jong Il, and Muammar Gaddafi.[40,41] Post has taught courses on personality and political behavior at the annual meetings of the American Psychiatric Association.

The website www.truthout.org has published several articles on the psychology and psychodynamics of Bush and Cheney written by a retired Westchester County (NY) psychiatrist (John Briggs) and his son John Briggs II (professor of journalism at Western Connecticut State University).[42,43] We spoke to both father and son (personal communication, April 14, 2008, and February 25, 2016), who received much positive commentary thanking the authors for providing some coherent descriptions and explanations of two public figures whom they thought had serious mental problems.

Frank Ochberg stated that, after watching video-tapes and reading the writings of Cho Seung Hui, who committed a mass shooting at Virginia Tech, he felt it his professional obligation to provide public education to a television and online blog audience who was being told that Cho was a "sociopath" similar to the Columbine high school killers seven years earlier.[44] Ochberg advanced the notion that Cho was "psychotic," not "sociopathic," and thought it important that the public understand the difference. Ochberg said he thought that psychiatrists, along with many other scientists, have abdicated their responsibilities to educate the public and to raise the level of debate in this country, and that the professional organization that represents psychiatry should encourage its members to engage in public discussions (personal communication April 4, 2008 and February 27, 2016).

We agree. Psychiatrists, as behavioral health specialists, have an obligation to help the community to understand public behaviors that do not match social standards and expectations. Psychiatrists have an obligation to share concerns about public figures who exhibit erratic or unprofessional behavior, as well as a need to help the public understand mass tragedies and acts of violence. Psychiatrists need to communicate that mental illness is illness, and that diagnostic terms are not epithets, even if some people misuse personality disorder terms such as "narcissistic," "borderline," and sociopathy as insults. Psychiatrists do not, on the other hand, have a moral obligation to make our profession look good in the public eye. We are not suggesting that psychiatrists should broadcast whatever ill-considered opinions they please in public forums in the name of psychiatry. Psychiatry is controversial in many circles, for myriad reasons, some better than others. To some, psychiatry has been and still is considered to be a political vehicle for controlling social unconventionality. Psychiatry has survived a 40-year unrelenting public attack by Thomas Szasz and others for this very charge of suppressing socially deviant behaviors; it will surely survive a few discomforting moments caused by problematic public comments by some members of our profession.[45,46]

We believe that the APA should attempt to set standards for the public behavior of its members. However, including the Goldwater Rule in the APA Code of Ethics gives it undue importance. Actions may be inadvisable and yet not sanctionable. The APA may engage in the same debates as do its members (and nonmember psychiatrists). To require individual psychiatrists to protect psychiatry's public image above their own competing values is both self-serving and misplaced. It is self-serving in that it may put the interests of the profession in direct conflict with the interests of well-meaning individual members. It is misplaced because it discourages rather than encourages public debate. In 1964, the participation of psychiatrists in the *Fact* magazine survey reflected poorly on the profession, but we cannot accuse those participants of acting wrongly so much as injudiciously. In this electronic age, when news and opinions travel faster and proliferate further than *Fact* ever did, public commentary is the norm and not the exception. Psychiatry should encourage scrutiny of the behaviors of public figures, not squelch it.

Conclusions

The Goldwater Rule is meant to direct psychiatrists from discrediting the profession by speaking falsely, irresponsibly, or with malice in the name of the profession. We have seen that despite its good intent, it contradicts regular psychiatric diagnostic practices, and its reach seems to include legitimate academic pursuits and self-promoting pseudoscientific statements by individual practitioners. The Goldwater Rule is redundant of sections of the professional ethics principles that protect patient privacy and promote public education, and it acknowledges that personal values may compete with professional obligations. We argue that the real purpose of the Goldwater Rule is to prevent individual psychiatrists from misrepresenting or embarrassing the psychiatric profession, possibly at the expense of personal, professional, or social values. We find this to be unreasonable. Psychiatrists have many social roles and identities, and it is inappropriate for the profession to expect that professional responsibilities will be prioritized in every instance. That is, professional standards of public conduct are important, but do not carry the moral weight of other psychiatric and personal values.

We can hope that psychiatrists who speak publicly about public figures will be thoughtful, scholarly, and non-contemptuous, and we can teach our trainees what constitutes good conduct. However, we cannot require psychiatrists to protect the profession's public image. To the extent that the Goldwater Rule inhibits potentially valuable educational efforts and psychiatric opinions about potentially dangerous public figures, upholding it is unethical. The court of public opinion will adjudicate professionalism and propriety, and the APA may opine in this setting, but embarrassing the profession violates etiquette rather than ethics.

Jerome Kroll, M.D., is Professor of Psychiatry Emeritus at the University of Minnesota Medical School. He has a B.A. (philosophy) from Brown University and an M.D. from Albert Einstein College of Medicine, and trained in psychiatry at Case Western Reserve University Hospitals. He served as Chief Psychiatrist for the Southeast Asian and East African Refugee Mental Health Program at the Community-University Health Care Clinic in Minneapolis (1978-2020) and presently works at a Somali-run clinic in Minneapolis. Dr. Kroll has written numerous books, including with Sir Martin Roth, The Reality of Mental Illness, *and with Bernard Bachrach,* The Mystic Mind.

Claire Pouncey, M.D., Ph,D., is a psychiatrist in private practice in Phil-adelphia, PA. She completed a combined M.D.-Ph.D. program in phi-losophy, focusing her graduate work on the philosophy of science. Her academic interests now include psychiatric epistemology, professional and psychiatric ethics, scientific classification, and explanation in psy-chedelic medicine. Her publications include the 2017 article, "President Trump's Mental Health—Is It Morally Permissible for Psychiatrists to Comment?" for the New England Journal of Medicine. *Dr. Pouncey is a past President of the Association for the Advancement of Philosophy and Psychiatry.*

References

1189 Psychiatrists Say Goldwater is Psychologically Unfit to be President. Fact Magazie, Vol 1, No. 5, 1964.

American Psychiatric Association: The Principles of Medical Ethics with Annotations Especially Applicable to Psychiatry. Washington, DC: American Psychiatric Association, 2009 Revised Edition.

Cooke BK, Goddard ER, Werner TL, et al: The risks and responsible roles for psychiatrists who interact with the media. J Am Acad Psychiatry Law 42:459–68, 2014.

Martin-Joy J: Images in psychiatry: Goldwater v. Ginzburg. Am J Psychiatry 2015: 172:729 –30, 2015.

Klitzman R: Should therapists analyze presidential candidates? New York Times Op-Ed Online, March 7, 2016. Available at http://nyti.ms/1Stp3YT. Accessed March 12, 2016.

Goldwater v. Ginzburg, 261 F. Supp. 784 (S.D.N.Y. 1966).

Goldwater v. Ginzburg, 414 F.2d 324 (2d Cir. 1969).

Ginzburg v. Goldwater, 396 U.S. 1049, (1970).

Ginzburg v. Goldwater, 396 U.S. 1049, 1054, (1970).

Sacks HS: POTUS and the Goldwater Rule. Psychiatric News, February 20, 1988. Available at http://psychnews.org/pnews/98-02-20/pres.html/. Accessed March 11, 2016.

Friedman RA: How a telescopic lens muddles psychiatric insights. New York Times, May 24, 2011, p D5.

Experts analyze Spitzer's thinking. Available at http://www.cnn.com/2008/LIVING/personal/03/11/spitzer/psychology.ap. Accessed April 6, 2008 (no longer available).

Reiss S: Does Eliot Spitzer have a normal personality? Available at http://www.cambridgeblog.org/2008/03/does-eliot-spitzer-havea-normal-personality/. Accessed April 6, 2008.

Friedman RA: Role of physicians and mental health professionals in discussions of public figures. JAMA 300:1348–50, 2008.

Friedman RA: The role of psychiatrists who write for popular media: experts, commentators, or educators? AmJ Psychiatry 166:757–9, 2009.

Post JM: Ethical considerations in psychiatric profiling of political figures. Psychiatr Clin North Am 25:635–46, 2002.

Kendell RE, Cooper JE, Gourlay AG: Diagnostic criteria of American and British psychiatrists. Arch Gen Psychiatry 25:123–30, 1971.

Cooper JE, Kendell RE, Gurland BJ, et al: Psychiatric diagnosis in New York and London. Maudsley Monograph No. 20. London: Oxford University Press, 1972.

Wing JK, Nixon J: Discriminating symptoms in schizophrenia: a report from the International Pilot Study of Schizophrenia. Arch Gen Psychiatry 32:853–9, 1975.

Freud S: A Case of Dementia Paranoides (Schreber Case), in Collected Papers, volume 3. New York: Basic Books, 1959.

Erikson E: Young Man Luther. New York: W. W. Norton, 1958.

Erikson E: Gandhi's Truth. New York: W. W Norton, 1969.

Mack JE: A Prince of our Disorder: Life of T.E. Lawrence. Cambridge: Harvard University Press, 1976.

Kroll J, DeGanck R: The adolescence of a thirteenth century visionary nun. Psychol Med 16:745–56, 1986.

Kroll J, DeGanck R: Beatrice of Nazareth: psychiatric perspectives on a medieval mystic. Cistercian Studies, 24:301–23, 1990.

Kroll J, Bachrach B: The Mystic Mind: The Psychology of Medieval Mystics and Ascetics. London: Routledge, 2005 pp 165–81.

Kroll J, Bachrach B: Justin's madness: weakmindedness or organic psychosis? J Hist Med 48:40–67, 1993.

Pouncey C: The psychiatrist in the community: a broader ethical perspective. Paper read at Symposium 85: APA's Goldwater Rule: Ethics of Speaking Publicly about Public Figures. American Psychiatric Association Annual Meeting, Washington,

DC, May 8, 2008.

Ablow K: Newt Gingrich's three marriages mean he might make a strong president—really. Available at: http://www.foxnews.com/opinion/2012/01/20. Accessed January 21, 2012.

Huffington Post: Keith Ablow, Fox News Psychiatrist: Newt Gingrich's infidelity might make him a better president. Available at http://www.huffingtonpost.com/2012/01/21/keith-ablow-foxnews-newt-gingrich-marriages_n_1220761.html. Accessed January 21, 2012.

Maza C: Meet Dr. Ablow, Fox News' Anti-LGBT Pop Psychologist. Equality Matters blog, September 26, 2011. Available at http://equalitymatters.org/blog/201109260010/. Accessed January 21, 2012.

Dr. Keith Abow: All wrong: in California girls can use urinals in boys' bathroom. January 14, 2014. Available at http://www.foxnews.com/opinion/2014/01/14/all-wrong-in-california-girlscan-use-urinals-in-boys-restroom.html. Accessed August 16, 2015.

Drescher J: Dr. Ablow gets it wrong about Chaz Bono and 'Dancing with the Stars. September 13, 2011. Available at http://www.foxnews.com/opinion/2011/09/13/dr-ablow-gets-it-wrongabout-chaz-bono-and-dancing-with-stars.html. Accessed June 4, 2015.

Glaad.org: Fox commentator's anti-trans claims are nonsense. Available at http://www.glaad.org/blog/fox-commentators-antitrans-claims-are-nonsense/. Accessed August 22, 2015.

Shore MF: How psychiatrists and political scientists have grown up since 1938. Psychiatry 64:192– 6, 2001.

Frank JA: Bush on the Couch: Inside the Mind of the President. New York: Harper, 2007.

Frank JA: Obama on the Couch: Inside the Mind of the President. New York: Free Press, 2011.

Frank JA: New York Times, letter to the Editor, Saturday March 12, 2016, p A18.

Dekleva KB, Post JM: Genocide in Bosnia: the case of Dr. Radovan Karadzic. J Am Acad Psychiatry Law 25:485–96, 1997.

Robins RS, Post JM: Political Paranoia: The Psychopolitics of Hatred. New Haven: Yale University Press, 1997.

Post JM: Leaders and Their Followers in a Dangerous World. Ithaca, NY: Cornell University Press, 2004.

John Briggs and John Briggs II: Bush and the psychology of incompetent decisions. Available at http://truth-out.org/archive/component/k2/item/68155:briggs-and-briggs–bush-and-thepsychology-of-incompetent-decisions/. Accessed January 18, 2007.

John Briggs and John Briggs II: Dick Cheney's Psychology: Part 2: The "Attendant Lord." Available at http://www.truth-out.org/archive/item/71788:dick-cheneys-psychology–part-2-theattendant-lord/. Accessed January 12, 2007.

Cullen D: Psychopath? Depressive? Schizophrenic? Was Cho SeungHui really like the Columbine killers? Posted Friday April 20, 2007. Available at www.slate.com/articles/health_and_science/medical_examiner/2007/04/psychopath_depressive_schizophrenic.html/. Accessed April 3, 2008.

Szasz TS: The Myth of Mental Illness. New York: Harper and Row, 1976.

Roth M, Kroll J: The Reality of Mental Illness. Cambridge, UK: Cambridge University Press, 1986 (reprinted 2009).

THE GOLDWATER RULE HOLDS NO WATER
—But Carries the Water for Oppression

RAVI CHANDRA, M.D.

> Allen Dyer, who served on the original commission that formulated the ethical principles applicable to psychiatrists, has noted that originally these were intended to be ethical principles, to serve as guidelines, where what is now referred to as the Goldwater Rule has become a prohibition in the sense of "Thou shalt not."
>
> Jerrold Post, M.D.,
> *Dangerous Charisma: The Political Psychology*
> *of Donald Trump and His Followers*

A lot has been written on the Goldwater Rule (GR) (Section 7.3 of the APA's Code of Ethics), including responses to Kroll and Pouncey's scholarly argument against it. I would say that of all that I've read, I haven't found anything that goes beyond reiterating the basic talking points that the APA has used for years, if not decades. These talking points are contestable, refutable, pure conjecture, and specious reasoning. The best you can say about them is that they are close-minded declarations made by those who are not experts in the field they opine about, and who arrogantly dismiss the professional opinions of experts in leadership, mass psychology, social and political psychology, and dangerousness.

What is striking is how their subjective opinion becomes black-and-white, incontrovertible reality, and how psychiatry is viewed both as having overwhelming power in a fragile culture, and is somehow also futile and fragile itself. It is interesting that we express our ambivalence as a split. We have not reconciled or accepted our ambivalences. We are split, suppressed or suppressors, and in tension.

At best, one might say it's better to be cautious and thorough rather than throw caution to the wind, but the Goldwater Rule draws itself into Moses-from-the-mountain-top, 11th-Commandment-level stature, and in my view becomes the Goldwater Gaslight, deluding us from thoughtful, genuine, honest inquiry in the public domain. Disagreement has turned into dissociation, in our association.

What began as a necessary but perhaps overreaching corrective to profession-al embarrassment in the 1960's has become a CYA for organizational psychiatry, with proven potential for suppressing freedom of thought and purging dissenters. Given the stakes of the next U.S. election, this is a dangerous spot to put organized psychiatry and some of its most valuable members. Under the guise of "playing it safe," the APA's GR is amplifying conditions for dangerousness, for psychiatrists and society-writ-large, and has become a conscious or unconscious tool of oppression.

Reason, compassion, and shared humanity are in great peril when ego and turf dominate. The APA thus far has displayed these all-too-human latter traits, which also make it a demoralizing, moribund and complicit actor in upholding an oppressive status quo. The status quo is an intellectualized, self-justifying, avoidant, do-and-say-nothing autocracy. Through its version of abstinence, the APA amplifies enactment over insight, setting up even responsible actors for persecution and pathologization by the "power player layer" of self-appointed priests and gatekeepers of the profession.

The APA has at best acquired and amplified a political phobia, fearing the politi-cization of psychiatry. However, silence and avoidance are also political acts. They inter-fere with collegial learning, and foreclose the possibility of psychiatry making a bigger difference in the life of the culture. They contribute to an atmosphere of *lèse majesté*, all for the "King's" benefit and the public's detriment, in a situation where, arguably, the Emperor has no clothes—or at least the public deserves full information to determine the extent of imperial couture.

The Goldwater Gaslight should be vacated, and psychiatrists freed to think and collaborate about supposedly "forbidden" and difficult subjects, while also being mem-bers of the APA, which remains the premier organization for the advancement of mental health in the nation, a mental health which will be further jeopardized under authoritarian and anti-democratic governmental control.

To my knowledge, there have been no referrals to the Ethics Committee for violations of the GR that have resulted in action. Because of the Constitution's First Amendment, no psychiatrist could be held legally liable for offering political, professional, personal, or even diagnostic opinions about political candidates or issues in the electorate, unless perhaps these opinions fell in the limited categories of unprotected speech, which would be adjudicated by a court of law.

Can the APA then state unequivocally what psychiatrists "can" or "should" say, regardless of First Amendment rights? Does the APA know, unequivocally, that it is not possible or desirable to offer professional opinions without direct interview and consent? Or is this an organizational preference that is in fact unfounded? Does the GR have a discourse-chilling or -killing effect that causes more harm than it is supposed to prevent?

In the current climate, it is not hard to see how the Goldwater Rule could be applied or misapplied by institutions such as universities or state medical boards to punish psychiatrists and other mental health practitioners for speaking their minds and expertise, when they run afoul of the political leanings, inhibitions, or phobias of those institutions. The GR can be used to ostracize and stigmatize psychiatrists utilizing their expertise as they best see fit. In fact, Dr. Bandy Lee has stated that the Yale Department of Psychiatry cited the Goldwater Rule in dismissing her from her faculty position, though she is not even a member of the APA.

Thus, the Goldwater Rule acts as a very concrete punitive superego, empowering some to become enforcers and guardians of "professionalism," and naysayers and deniers of other trained psychiatrists' professional opinions and observations. This especially affects and afflicts minoritized physicians who are historically more likely to speak out in times of political oppression and dangerousness, and in any case are more affected by those times. The GR infantilizes professionals, and assumes they cannot assess the risks of offering professional opinions themselves, or that they would knowingly stigmatize those with mental illness, and that their professional opinions would be no more than mere name-calling, grandstanding, and evidence of their own political biases and grandiosity, bringing disrepute to the profession and creating mistrust. At best, it fights the war of the 1960's *Fact Magazine* controversy, without seeing the battlefield before us today.

The Goldwater Rule has also likely placed a muzzle on political discourse within the body of the APA. Word-of-mouth has it that there was a significant exodus of members from the APA in 2016-17 precisely because the APA was unwilling to bend on the GR. Word-of-mouth also has it that there was active discrimination against topics deemed "too political" at the election year 2024 APA Annual Meeting in New York City.

This mental-muzzle (or psychic straightjacket) has prevented the membership from learning about and grappling with the effects of politics and political leadership on our patients and ourselves. We are in uncharted territory with disinformation and the astonishing rise of threats of political violence and antagonism to democracy. Psychiatrists, and the APA membership, seem to be relatively uninformed about the effects of political leaders and their behaviors and statements on mental health, and because of the GR, unable to "connect the dots" from those behaviors to responsible risk assessments of leaders and political movements on vulnerable populations or the institutions of democracy writ large.

In the past, the APA has worked to educate members about the effects of authoritarian leaders and means of social control. In 1989, the APA published Dr. Marc Galanter's book *Cults and New Religious Movements*, which included a chapter on cult leadership. In that chapter, Dr. Alexander Deutsch wrote:

I will attempt to explain the power and attraction of the cult leader. I will describe and analyze the paradoxical adherence of certain devotees to their leaders in the face of facts which should logically lead to disillusionment. In the last section, I will describe how devotees of a psychotic leader can become pawns for the acting out of the leader's bizarre inner conflicts…

What benefits accrue to a psychotic or pre-psychotic leader from having a devoted following? What are the bonds that tie such an individual to his or her group?

In a section entitled "The Psychotic Cult Leader" he writes:

A "worst case" example of blind obedience of cult members is provided by the mass suicide and murder in Jonestown, Guyana, in 1978. Jim Jones, the leader, in a state of paranoid deterioration, instigated the apocalyptic ending of the People's Temple. For many years prior to the massacre, while doing "good deeds" like helping the poor and preaching interracial harmony, there were signs of megalomania and paranoia in the leader.

Psychiatrist Robert Jay Lifton, a founder of the field of psychohistory, is well known for his analysis of "thought reform." He analyzed (from a distance and without their consent) individuals and groups who committed war crimes.

Dr. Jerrold Post founded the program in political psychology at George Washington University and the Center for the Analysis of Personality and Political Behavior at the CIA. When his risk analysis of Saddam Hussein went public in Congressional testimony, he was called before the APA Ethics Committee for possible violation of the GR. He responded, and never heard from them again.

These are all examples of "professional and diagnostic opinions" which seem to be forbidden (or at least called into question) by the Goldwater Rule, yet they all arguably provided knowledge and wisdom for social well-being.

Indeed, the GR appears to be quite ambivalent and inconclusive on what psychiatrists "can" and "can't" say. For example, on page 106 of the 2024 Opinions of the Ethics Committee on The Principles of Medical Ethics:

> Yet, nothing in the clarification prohibits psychiatrists from exercising their rights to speak as private citizens or to comment in general about the implications of certain publicly observed behaviors and the potential psychiatric implications of such behaviors. It is the difference between professional and personal opinions that matters here, as well as the specificity of the response.

The APA might as well report that this area is highly subjective. What, precisely, is the boundary between "professional" and "personal" opinion, when you are talking about "potential psychiatric implications" of a public figure's behavior and personality? What if my opinion is derived from an exploration of political and social psychology, and my professional expertise? What if I comment on psychological defenses and how these might suggest character or personality traits? What if I examine publicly available data to give a humble opinion on cognitive, empathic, or relational capacity? Wouldn't the public likely benefit from such informed opinion? How might any of this differ from what Post, Lifton, Deutsch, or Galanter offered?

Dr. Charles Dike recently wrote in *Psychiatric News*, reiterating the talking points mentioned earlier, that violations of the GR could "result in a degradation of trust in psychiatrists" and that "psychiatrists should always be acutely aware that their public pronouncements have the potential to strip individuals of their humanity, dignity, and respect. Such power demands the highest degree of responsibility, accountability, and restraint.

With all due respect to Dr. Dike, this is a quite paternalistic statement, and is wholly unsupported. He suggests that offering professional opinions "could result in a degradation of trust"— but there's no evidence for this. It is at least as likely that not offering professional opinions about leaders could result in a degradation of trust in the APA and the profession more broadly, especially amongst the most vulnerable populations.

Whose trust in us will be degraded if we opine about, say, malignant narcissism and dangerousness of a political candidate? Could it be the dominant and dominating culture that expects us to stay in line and be silent, when they threaten BIPOC, LGBTQ, women, the disabled, and so forth? Could it be the dominant culture of an ancient version of psychoanalysis, which demands "neutrality" and "abstinence? Why has the APA become both more strident and perhaps more ambivalent about the GR since 2017? I might suggest that our times are the "exception that probes the rule," and the APA's gymnastics on this issue represent a culture under difficult conditions of stress and change. As we all know, resistance to input and change is to be expected under such circumstances.

But whose humanity, dignity, and respect is actually being stripped, as we speak of prohibiting comments on clear and present dangers in a thoughtful, well-reasoned manner?

In fact, the APA did sponsor an APA TV video which directly implicated Donald Trump in mental health impacts of COVID-19 on Asian American mental health. Where is the line between personal and professional opinion? Is there one? The APA seems to be ambivalent, and hedges its bets in different directions, yet the most visible output is the reiteration of the Goldwater rule as stricture and means of control.

The DSM-V-TR states that "[r]acism exists at personal, interpersonal, systemic/institutional, and social structural level," and "[negative racial stereotypes and attitudes affect the psychological development and well-being of racialized groups."

Is it not incumbent upon concerned psychiatrists to not only point out the racism (and sexism, homophobia, transphobia, etc.) of political leaders, but help members and the general public "connect the dots" to psychological defenses, techniques of propaganda and manipulation, and character and risk analysis? Given our times, if autocratic political forces are further emboldened and empowered, these passages in our own DSM will come under great scrutiny and pressure— precisely as a function of the racism we are trying to overcome. Will these passages be labeled "discriminatory" or "critical race theory" by the far-right? Our medico-political speech, including this speech in the DSM, is in defense of our patients and our own organization's thinking capacity.

Instead, the APA is an umpire that officially calls our professional wisdom "out of bounds" and "unprofessional," while perhaps tacitly approving of our work. As a minoritized psychiatrist, I am well aware that accusations of unprofessionalism have been used to marginalize the emotions and perspectives of the oppressed, when in fact oppression creates distressing emotions and alternate perspectives. The GR is thus a tool of oppression, make no mistake, by silencing those most knowledgeable and most afflicted or in compassionate allyship with those most afflicted, and preventing psychiatrists from learning about pressing matters in support of patient care and society.

Perhaps the GR provides an effective legal and cultural shield for the APA, but it throws our profession into dissociation and cognitive dissonance, as a fixed idea of dubious merit but boundless and even ruthless application.

Again, whom does it benefit to authoritatively state psychiatrists "should not" or "cannot" make diagnoses or professional opinions without personal evaluation and consent? Doesn't psychiatry's great advance lie in the capacity to recognize and call forth suppressed content—not to further suppress and repress?

Dr. Dike also acknowledges that psychiatrists offer opinions in legal and other contexts without personal examination, but he allows that these:

> psychiatrists are still required to review all relevant documents and obtain
> corroborative information by interviewing relevant parties. Without these
> activities, the objectivity of a psychiatrist's opinion would appropriately
> be called into question.

How is this any different from reviewing the massive amount of publicly available information about President Trump, including his public statements, and reports of behavior that have come out in numerous memoirs, and perhaps interviewing those directly or indirectly impacted by him?

And what is wrong with having one's objectivity called into question? Shouldn't we welcome such questioning, and be able to answer it? The days of the "blank screen" analyst are long behind us. We all may have biases, and the best among us work hard to minimize bias in service of our patients, and enter into relationship with them with full humility and humanity. This is certainly possible as we consider offering our professional opinions in the public sphere.

There are those who might say, "Well, we are not in therapeutic relationship with public figures." Actually, both public figures and psychiatrists working in the public field are in relationship with society, and society emerges out of countless interactions of individuals and groups. In the Lakota saying, *mitakuye oyasin*. We are all related. We must be allowed to relate fully, with insight, compassion, and thoughtfulness. Society keeps the score of our traumatic dissociations. Psychiatry can play a role in creative reintegration by propagating thoughtful, compassionate discussion of leaders' vulnerabilities, strengths, and potential dangerousness.

Also, it should be noted that psychiatrists are often required to make diagnoses and offer professional opinions based on written or video vignettes, for example for Board certification. And we routinely offer analysis and insight on people in our patients' social milieu, for the benefit of our patients. So, the idea that we "cannot" make such distinctions is false on the very face. The APA's injunction that we "should not" is highly questionable, and as I've said, in support of the dominant culture's enterprise against accountability and insight, and in support of outmoded and questionable psychoanalytic principles.

Thus, it appears the main (perhaps unstated) arguments for the GR are to avoid controversy and "jeopardy" for the APA, especially in its governmental relations.

We should be reminded, as I close, of how psychiatry was complicit in stigmatizing gays and lesbians in this century, and how it authoritatively labeled Blacks running away from slavery as insane.

As the ACT UP activists told us in the 1980's: Silence = Death.

Perhaps the most succinct interpretation of the Goldwater Rule is: "The Truth is Out There: Let's Hide!"

The GR is a slogan, dogma, a religious mantra, a shibboleth, an article of fundamentalist faith, the pablum of the heretofore ruling class of psychiatry, and the opiate of the medical masses, and through them, the population as a whole. Or to use philosopher Harry Frankfurt's terminology, "Bullshit."

Ravi Chandra, M.D., is a psychiatrist, writer, and compassion educator in San Francisco, and a Distinguished Fellow of the American Psychiatric

Association. He received an Sc.B. with Honors from Brown University, an M.D. from Stanford University School of Medicine, and completed a residency in general adult psychiatry from the University of California, San Francisco. He writes for Psychology Today *and* East Wind eZine. *His debut nonfiction book,* Facebuddha: Transcendence in the Age of Social Networks, *won a 2017 Nautilus Silver Award. His debut documentary feature, "The Bandaged Place: From AIDS to COVID and Racial Justice," was awarded Best Film at the 2021 Cannes Independent Film Festival.*

References

American Psychiatric Association. (2024 Edition) Opinions of the ethics committee on the principles of medical ethics.

APA TV on YouTube. (2021, April 23). Asian-American mental health during COVID-19. (video sponsored by APA).

Byman, D. L (2021, April 9). Commentary: How hateful rhetoric connects to real-world violence. Brookings Institution.

Chandra, R. (2024, May 19). Responsible dialogue on the "Goldwater rule" must continue. *Psychology Today*.

Dike, C. (2024, March 25). As another election looms, the Goldwater rule remains relevant as ever. *Psychiatric News*.

Frankfurt, H. (2005). On bullshit. Princeton University Press.

Hahamy, M., & Horta, B. (2024, January 23). Former professor says Yale fired her over tweet on Trump, Dershowitz. *Yale Daily News*, X

Kroll, J., & Pouncey, C. (2016, June). The Ethics of the Goldwater Rule. *JAAPL*, online 44 (2) (pp. 226-235).

Mahdanian, A. A., & Rosen, A., et al. (2024, January 23). A call to avoid psychiatric labelling in a historic election year. *The Lancet Psychiatry,* Vol 11 (3): (pp.168–169).

Woolhandler, S., & Himmelstein, D. U., et al. (2021, February 21). Public policy and health in the Trump era. *The Lancet*.

THE CHALLENGE OF WRITING ABOUT DONALD TRUMP IN 2017

Henry J. Friedman M.D.

The challenge for a psychiatrist like myself, in writing critically about Donald Trump in 2017, came from the American Psychiatric Association's Goldwater Rule, with its insistence that, as a psychiatrist, I was prevented from commenting on the mental health of any public figure whom I had not examined in person. To do so was to risk at least the disapproval of that organization, and at most, being expelled from it. From the beginning I felt there was something wrong with this stance when it came to commenting on Donald Trump and the nature of his pathological character. My first thought was that I had seen more of Trump on television and could tell more about him than any in-person interview with him as a patient would allow me to do. The observations that I had made of him during his successful 2016 campaign convinced me that his was a most dangerous personality type. Commenting on his character didn't feel to me like making a diagnosis as much as offering a description informed by my psychiatric experience about a man in a unique position. Indeed, Trump did somehow convince a significant part of the population that he would solve their problems, make their lives better, and in fact, transform America into something which could be called, in his terms, "great again". What I had seen in observing Donald Trump on his many television appearances had convinced me that he was paranoid, grandiose, and a would-be dictator; a prediction that was proven correct when he attempted to subvert the peaceful transfer of power following his clear defeat in the 2020 election. The paranoid core of his personality was revealed in his unswerving belief in nonexistent dangers that threatened this country, and his belief that the United States was in a state of carnage and decay. This kind of exaggerated appraisal of danger and where it resided seems so clearly the thinking of dictators that have come

149

before him, and constitutes evidence of his essential totalitarian orientation towards the country and its citizens.

During the four years of his presidency, observations that confirmed my impression were possible and plentiful. He degraded and threatened anyone who opposed him, and was completely shut off from learning from others anything about himself or the world he was living in. All of this was made even more obvious after the COVID-19 pandemic began to engulf our country. President Trump insisted on inserting himself at the front and center of press conferences about the pandemic; thereby, contributing further evidence of his paranoid relationship to the world. The Chinese had to be blamed for creating a virus and exporting it to our country. He seemed to be at war with science, and approached the pandemic more as a challenge to his omnipotence than to a devastating disease that was killing hundreds of thousands of people. His main concern seemed to be established around proving his omnipotence in the name of his ability to get rid of this virus. The memorable meeting in which he described his wish to eliminate it using disinfectant that could wipe it out completely, demonstrated a mind that was dominated by solipsistic thinking and paranoid grandiosity. Somehow, he became convinced that masks were the enemy of the people, instead of acknowledging that we had to do everything possible to protect ourselves from a deadly virus. He turned against his medical advisers, insisting they were wrong about both masks and the need to self-isolate. When he himself became seriously ill with COVID-19, he attempted to ignore it, and then to give the impression that his strength of character had made it possible for him to overcome the virus. This concentration on his power to control even a virus that had invaded his body should have alerted the public to his mental incompetency; but, as was to be proven over and over again, he managed to shake off what should have been conclusive evidence that he was unfit to serve as President of the United States. His preoccupation with power and size of crowds were manifestations of his desire to be a dictator. His admiration for totalitarian leaders reflected his desire to have the kind of power they had in the countries they ruled.

I had never imagined seeing an American president who was not to be trusted to follow the constitution and protect us from violations of personal safety. He manifested a complete ignorance of the Cold War and the history of Russia as our enemy, even to the extent of denying U.S. intelligence on Russian interference in the 2016 election, preferring instead to favor Putin's assertions.

The nature of Trump as a dictator (as is the case with dictatorships wherever they exist) meant that he would become increasingly brutal in response to challenges to his grandiosity. His preoccupation with those seeking asylum by crossing our southern border escalated into the policy of separating children from their parents, thereby discouraging refugees from entering the United States. Again, under the influence of his paranoid nature, these refugees were seen as dangerous criminals and mentally ill individuals, who only sought to enter the country to commit crimes and rapes. Paradoxically, the policy of separating children from the parents indicated that many, if not most, of the refugees seeking asylum were families hoping to protect their children; instead, these parents found their children taken away in a totally devastating fashion. At that time, the parent-child separation cruelty seemed to suggest Trump had the potential to abut Hitler and his policies of murdering children and their parents to satisfy his obsession with Jews, and his uncontrollable desire to rid Europe of all Jews. This did not happen with Trump during his presidency, but it does suggest possible future actions on his part, should he be elected again and given the power to act on his instincts and impulses with all their desire to destroy and eliminate his enemies.

The possibility that his grandiosity would prevent him from accepting defeat in the election of 2020 was predictable, even expectable. His disdain for President Biden was such that it prevented him from even considering the possibility that he had been defeated. He needed to believe otherwise not because he was vulnerable, but because he could not conceive of the idea that somebody he viewed as inferior and as a loser could in fact legitimately win an election against him. It was obvious to me that he was not going to leave office and allow for the peaceful transfer of power that our national elections had always permitted. Instead, he indulged paranoid fantasies that the election machines were tampered with and that election workers threw out ballots that were for him. He was so convinced of this fact that he encouraged and promoted a mob to attack the Capitol on January 6, 2021. There should be no doubt that his intentions were lethal, that he would have allowed the mob to kill many of our leaders if he believed that he could successfully retain the position of president. I think we have all minimized how close it really was to a coup that would have given him what he wanted—the ability to continue as president despite having lost the election.

Insight into paranoid grandiosity as a character should protect us from assumptions that Trump is like a child. This kind of assertion has been common in the media and it is woefully inadequate. Trump's dangerous nature has nothing to do with his childish behavior or so-called narcissistic personality. Narcissism has nothing to do with paranoid grandiosity; it is a kind of character that is self-centered but of a different kind of self-centeredness than what we see in Donald Trump. Narcissistic personalities are not dangerous; they may make those around them—their spouse, their children—unhappy, even miserable, but there is nothing to indicate they have the capacity or the desire for dictatorial power. When I first suggested that Trump was an American Hitler, many people objected that this went too far. More than ever, I am convinced that my assertion about the parallels between Trump and Hitler are eerily accurate. Like Hitler, Trump, in his grandiose effort to make America great again, will be capable of allowing Putin to re-annex the Ukraine, and making alliances with Putin to take the United States out of NATO. This would allow Russia to regain its satellite states, all of whom would be prey to Putin's expansionism without the United States military to back them up. His plans are outlined in the document Project 2025, a 900-page outline of the plan for a second Trump term. Trump insists that he has not approved of Project 2025, but it has his stamp all over it (and was written by a coalition of his former staffers.) Among other concerning agenda items, it aims to make certain that abortion is declared illegal for the entire nation.

We need to think about Trump's paranoid preoccupation with immigrants as very much the equivalent of Hitler's preoccupation with Jews. The need to cleanse the country of illegal immigrants is parallel to Hitler's need to eliminate the Jews of Europe to purify and protect the continent. Does this sound extreme? Not if you really think about the plan to round up millions of illegal and legal immigrants and deport them. It should be remembered that Hitler's initial plan was based upon the idea of expelling the Jews, putting them into concentration camps and then deporting them; when no one would take them he developed the Final Solution. Are we going to see a Final Solution coming from Trump and his followers? In the end, he will deport millions of people. Perhaps we do differ from the Weimar republic in the 1920's in that our economy is not a disaster, nor is the nation filled with carnage. But have no illusion that Trump will restrain himself from insisting this is the case, and that many will believe they need protection from immigrants, among other vaguely defined enemies. It is easy to imagine what another four years of Trump would allow him to do to this nation. I have little doubt that we would end up as Germany did, a broken nation, due to his destructive impulses. It was easy for establishment figures in Germany to write off Hitler as a populist phenomenon that could be controlled once he assumed power. They believed he would be a passing leader—and millions of people died because of that erroneous belief.

Recently I was talking with a 94-year-old patient of mine who is a lifetime Republican. When he mentioned that he was going to vote for Trump, I asked him how he felt about Trump's unpleasant language and threatening tone, both of which were so different from anything I had ever heard from my patient. He agreed that those aspects of what he heard from Trump were distressing. So why, I asked, are you still voting for him? His answer: Trump is strong and he will keep us safe. I didn't bother to ask further about *what* he would keep us safe from; and yet, my patient volunteered that the immigrants coming over the border were a distinct danger to him, even though he lived in the Northeast far from any urban center. I found what he described as informative and terrifying. The idea that this pathological individual, with his talent for cruelty and dictatorship, would once again hold the seat of power because he could convince enough voters that he was strong in a positive sense is deeply alarming. The notion that he can protect us is a lie that could morph into the kind of bigger lie that convinces people to condemn themselves to totalitarian leadership. The loss of democracy that is based upon free elections has never seemed more possible than it does now. There are conmen and sociopaths that we encounter on a personal level in life; they cause injuries and distress for those in contact with them, but this cannot be confused with what someone with a dictatorial character can produce in any nation where they achieve power. That power rarely is applied for the good of the people; primarily it is wielded for the gratification of the dictator, for his delight in having the ability to inflict pain and suffering on those who oppose him. While there is hope that Trump will lose the upcoming election, there is also the possibility that the public will be fooled again, that as a result of the electoral college he will be victorious. Our future rests on the outcome of this election, and that outcome should be based upon the dangerousness of Donald Trump as has been described by several psychiatrists and mental health workers in this volume. If he wins, we can forget about anything resembling free and fair elections; he will be above the law and he will be our Hitler.

If in the end Trump is defeated in the election of 2024, it will go a long way towards reducing his impact on American culture. But it is important to remember that he has already coarsened acceptable public political dialogue. His impact will not fade until long after he is defeated, dead and gone. The reason for this is that he has already been able to win people over to a form of violence in speech, and advocated in action impulsive destructivity, something which his predecessors had uniformly managed to move away from. How is it possible that one man, equipped only with speech and hate speech at that, could have captured the minds of so many US citizens? The vulnerability of the electorate is a result of the widespread presence of paranoid personalities in our country.

The belief in the danger of the other, in both their inferiority and yet the other's danger appeals to the paranoid personality. Richard Hofstetter wrote about paranoia in American politics; he essentially describes this vulnerability as: The wish to believe that somebody who is black or Jewish or gay has the power to contaminate society and dislodge it from its perfection merely by existing. It is important to remember that the media, with its ability to reach into the homes of all citizens, can become a conduit for the spread of a new way of condoning violent "patrons" of those who are different. On the other hand, as we have seen, the media can also provide the most potent antidote to allowing the degradation of standards in American politics. Like most psychiatrists I know, we are eager for a positive outcome, in which the openly destructive qualities Trump has brought to life will fade and die, rather than simply go underground, only to re-emerge when the next would-be dictator arrives on the scene. As a divided country, we can only hope the division will be reduced on the side of the decent and good, rather than on the side of the brutal and evil, but we will all have to wait and see what happens in November and in the crucial months that follow the election.

Henry J. Friedman is a psychiatrist and psychoanalyst who trained in medicine at the Johns Hopkins School of Medicine, and in psychiatry at Harvard Medical School. He has been in the private practice of psychoanalysis and analytic psychotherapy since 1980, and has been an associate professor of psychiatry at both Tufts and Harvard Medical Schools. His main focus has been on the need for critical reappraisal of psychoanalytic theory and technique, especially the incompatibilities involved in different psychoanalytic theories and the failure to question basic assumptions. He has reviewed over 70 psychoanalytic books from an independent critical perspective.

EIGHT YEARS LATER

HOWARD H. COVITZ PH.D.

Don't you love farce?
My fault, I fear
I thought that you'd want what I want
Sorry, my dear!
But where are the clowns
Send in the clowns
Don't bother, they're here.
                    Stephen Sondheim, 1973

It was almost eight years ago, soon after the 2016 U.S. elections, that Bandy Lee put out a call for chapters to a proposed volume on the dangerousness of having Donald Trump occupy the presidency of the United States and the *de facto* leadership of the Free World. The broadly constituted nations of that Free World embrace a variety of democratic forms of governance and a similar variation in the forms that equal protection under law takes in those nations. They were and are the nations that successfully grew away from monarchies and autocracies and various forms of dictatorship. We tend to forget how much of the world was governed autocratically one hundred years ago and before. There were no such constitutional democracies 250 years ago. And it was less than 150 years prior that King Charles was convicted of treason and executed (30 January 1649) outside the Banqueting House in Whitehall for *crimes against the state*. The birth pangs of democracy's birth kept coming, as the World sought more egalitarian forms of living.

The twenty-seven (thirty-seven in the second edition) contributors to Lee's edited volume were mental health professionals, the individuals to whom an ethical and, in many U.S. States, a legal responsibility falls to warn about people who, due to their thinking and/or behaviors, are a risk to causing significant damage to themselves and/or to others. We, the authors were not focused upon diagnosis, recognizing that free countries do not forcibly segregate anyone from the population, nor do they restrict activities or rights based upon a psychological diagnosis but rather we choose to separate people or restrict some of their rights due to our recognition of the dangerousness they pose to self or others.

In consideration of these concerns, I chose to focus in the Lee volume upon two matters. The first was in the form of a question: Did I, as a clinical psychologist and a psychoanalyst, have a right to offer such judgments regarding *the fitness to serve* of a man I had never met and who, furthermore, had not granted me the right to talk about him publicly? Formally, as I was not a psychiatrist, I was not bound by the ethical standards set by the Goldwater Rule. Still, there were both contemporary and historical rules and laws of confidentiality—the sacred part of the therapeutic contract—that were to be breached, if ever, only in situations where there was a clear and present danger to others to which my silence would effectively contribute. I began the chapter in Lee's volume (Lee, 2017), indeed, citing a singular sentence in Leviticus XIX (written well over 2,000 years ago), whose existence demonstrated to me that this tension between Confidentiality and the Duty to Warn could not be considered a modern construction, "Don't go loose-lipped among your people (but) don't stand idly by as your neighbor bleeds; I am God," the writer of Leviticus commanded. My conclusion, effectively, was that the Goldwater Rule, like any other regulation, could only be understood fully with a list of the exceptional circumstances that might vitiate the general rule. It was, therefore, both as a citizen and as a seasoned mental health professional that I decided the Goldwater Rule was rightly trumped by my Duty to Warn others of the dangers that I saw in having Trump as president and that I see at least as clearly, today.

Secondly, and having made the decision that I was confronted by a situation exceptional to the Goldwater Rule, I outlined the six characteristics that I saw manifest in Trump's behavior that—in my clinical judgment—together made him: unfit to serve as president; a danger to the Republic; and a danger to its citizens and, potentially, to others. I reported seeing in Donald Trump's overt behavior and speech the characteristics of severely personality-disordered people who are likely to pose a threat to the general welfare. I left open the possibility that Trump was—*qua* entertainer—simply putting on a show. I did not know then and I cannot know now whether his behaviors are or were performative, a form of performance art but, then again, I concluded that a person who intentionally acts in these ways has opened himself up to the observer's conclusions. I repeat here the six cascading characteristics of such dangerously personality-disordered people (Covitz, 2017):

1. Such people are generally incapable of understanding and responding in an emotionally empathic way to how another feels, treating others as objects to be used rather than subjects in their own right.

2. Black-and-white thinking effectively splits the person's perceived world into those who support him and all those others who are against him….

3. Lacking the need to evaluate how their actions may impact others, these people react more quickly and with less skepticism about the correctness of their actions….

4. Such individuals have not developed a respect for others' thinking, relationships, or efforts. They ignore the necessity for maintaining extant organizations, government structures, conventional practices, laws, and alliances between others and between other nations.

5. Due to the above (1-4), their thinking is focused but lacks nuance….

6. Finally, (following on 1-5, above) they display a limited capacity to distinguish the real from the wished-for or imagined.

Trump demonstrated the good-fit of these six characteristics to his behaviors as president, ex-president, and presidential candidate. He attacked, mocked and demonized others and other groups (1 and 2). He acted rashly and often without concern for life during the pandemic and on the January 6th attack on the Capitol (3). He attacked anyone in power—including judges and witnesses and legislators—who confronted him. He apologized to no one and no nation, posted incompetents and foreign agents to critical positions within his administration and vitiated or threatened protective international alliances and historically important partnerships (4). And he continued to preference solely his own thinking at any given moment, independent of its truth value or what he may have said before (5 and 6). Many others have in this volume and elsewhere offered particular instances of each of these (1-6), and I will not repeat them here. What I will offer is a certain hypothesis that I posited in a later note (Covitz, 2020) at the end of Trump's *lengthy* four-year presidency and that I maintain, to this day.

Still, I can hardly do other than admire Trump's success in winning the fealty of nearly half the voting population of the United States. After all, he had none of the expectable *bona fides*. He had no successful experiences leading large governments or corporations. He wouldn't show the voters his tax returns that might demonstrate some legal and successful trajectory in life. He had been accused of a multitude of sexual peccadilloes and more serious sexual crimes. Trump was unlike any candidate who had ever arisen before him. He was, that is, not "presidential" and yet was chosen by over 70 million voters and carried the Electoral College, even if he lost the popular vote.

How did he do it? Whether he was borrowing from previous temporarily-successful despots or innovating all on his own, his methods were and are quite successful, specifically in garnering support from what was once the conservative half of the American electorate and their chosen leaders. (Aside: these were often the very same leaders who lambasted President Obama for wearing a summer-colored suit!) The very fact that the Religious Right in the United States has embraced the kind of man they would likely refuse to trust with their wallets, souls, or daughters speaks of some unconscious group process that, I suspect, sociologists and psychologists will explore for centuries. Consider just one such example of the madness under which we have lived: Mr. Trump managed to take the Republican Party from a broadly anti-Russian bloc to one that speaks in glowing terms of the likes of Vladimir Putin and Viktor Orbán!

The would-be Dictator in a democratic republic must come to control a critical mass of the people who are willing to follow him—no matter what—and to fight for him. He must overcome whatever sense these people have, as Americans, that investing too much power in a single person does not cohere well with democratic principles. The United States has, indeed, watched as legislators from both Houses of government, after being berated and—not infrequently—having their spouses and family disparaged, have come to Trump as supplicants, signing on to fully support him—kissing *his* ring and embracing each other, as if they comprised a homogeneous group of religious devotees— which they empirically do not.

Le Bon (1895) had already raised such questions of *how* such allegiances form in his treatise on *The Crowd*, concluding that a type of hypnotic trance brought together diverse actors who would then do things together and in a group that they would not ordinarily do as individuals. Freud (1921) had his own reasons for specific disagreements with Le Bon but in essence agreed that a certain hypnotic transference to a *muscular leader* or ideal is the secret sauce that permits the Leader to take control of the masses.

After five years of living—as most of us have—under the daily barrage of what became, so to speak, Trump TV, with its daily announcement of what Trump did or was accused of having done or what he said, I offered the following simple hypothesis (Covitz, 2020):

> The Leader who seeks imperial power effectively creates an outrageous persona that with certain differences will be taken on by not only those who support him but also unwittingly by those who oppose him. The outrageousness is fundamental to his strategy, whether the Leader recognizes the centrality of this outrageousness to accomplish complete domination of the nation he seeks to control.

The would-be despot (almost always male) chooses an outrageously stylized way of being, one that is identifiably unique and that will certainly be opposed by a majority of the people that find his style over-the-top, offensive, and opposed to the common good. They think of him initially and before he rises to power as a Clown—a sympathetic figure who surprises one and all with occasional naughtiness or evil. The Leader identifies the members of this majority as enemies of the people. He has previously identified a sizable minority of the people (in the neighborhood of 30-40%) who might well tolerate his outrageous behaviors, in no small part because they see the majority as oppressing them and him as successfully opposing that majority. He tells them that he and he alone—though mercilessly oppressed, himself, by that same majority—can free them from their pain caused by that majority. They are promised a wonderful world that he alone can provide. He mobilizes and agitates the now-angry minority while telling them that he—again, he and only he—can save them from the oppression of that malevolent majority.

This hypothesized process is self-sustaining, through the Leader's frequent use of violent-near rhetoric that renders (and is intended to render) the now no-longer-silent

159

minority angry, thus threatening the majority that, itself, has now been forced to admit its own hatred for the Clown. He tells his people, "I am your retribution ... they are coming after you." The Clown has by now risen in stature to someone of great power while the opposing majority—like the group of Good Germans in the late 1930's—maintains a subdued level of hateful thought and becomes inured—if frightened—to the raised levels of tension in this new World.

When a democratic republic begins to show cracking in its foundational documents, or when someone or some movement intentionally induces a constitutional crisis in that Republic for their own purposes, the mental health professional community in a democratic republic can do little more than make themselves available to offer commentary on the potential dangerousness of those who would split the country into warring factions for their own emotional and personal gain—we can, in the end, do little else than warn about and report our findings. No small thing!

Howard H. Covitz, Ph.D., A.B.P.P., has combined the practice of psychoanalysis in the suburbs of Philadelphia with a variety of other interests. He has taught university-level mathematics, psychology, and biblical characterology (1968–2011), was a training analyst at the Institute for Psychoanalytic Studies and the Institute for Psychoanalytic Psychotherapies, and its director (1986–98). He also ran a school for disturbed inner-city adolescents in the 1970's. His Oedipal Paradigms in Collision *(1998, reissued in 2016) was nominated for the Gradiva Book of the Year Award. His connectedness to his wife, grown children, and grandchildren motivates his writing and thinking.*

SEVEN YEARS LATER

Leonard L. Glass, M.D., M.P.H.

Looking back on 2017, the date *The Dangerous Case of Donald Trump*[1] was published, provides an opportunity for reflection. What did that book and similar writings by mental health professionals accomplish, if anything? Was it necessary? Ethical? Useful? Responsible? Damaging to the field, its authors, and patients seeking unbiased professional mental health care? All of these questions were raised pointedly at the time.[2,3,4,5]

Seven years later we approach another election in which Mr. Trump is the candidate of one of our two major political parties, and enjoys a following of nearly half the voting population. Here we are again. What can be fairly said about our early and repeated efforts to alert the public to the dangers we believed Trump carried if he won the presidency?

[I do recognize that I am not the most unquestionably neutral person to offer an assessment, given my contribution to *The Dangerous Case* book[6] and subsequent writings, but I will try to bear that handicap in mind below.]

Did our writings raise awareness of Trump's psychological aberrations?

In a way this is the lowest bar—it is almost impossible to see Trump in action and not recognize he is an unusual person. Indeed, many are drawn to him because he doesn't present as a traditional politician. But our task was to point out that his extraordinary personality was more than refreshing, entertaining, and gutsy, but harbored critical dangers to the country's values and well-being.

I would answer this question in three ways:

(1) The meteoric sales of *The Dangerous Case* to near the top of the New York

Times and Amazon best-seller lists indicated a widespread interest in learning what mental health workers made of Trump's aberrant behavior. Even if we were read with skepticism, our analyses gained traction in the public discourse.

(2) I don't think our reasoning made a dent in the adherence of the MAGA faithful. While much has been written about why so many cling to Mr. Trump as a credible leader, and even savior, despite the "Access Hollywood" tape[7]; his obvious lying; felony convictions; impeachments; AND our professional observations; that loyalty seems impervious to our efforts at what we saw as enlightenment.

(3) Using the barometer of the New York Times' editorial board as an imperfect gauge of the middle ground of public opinion, I do think we've gotten through. Initially the Times editorially reproached Bandy Lee (the editor), *et al.*, for publishing material in violation of Goldwater.[8] But over the course of seven years' time, the Times has virtually used our language (without attribution, I must add) in their consensus editorials, and published our letters sharing our view that Donald Trump is psychologically unfit to serve as president.[9] The left-leaning but still venerable *Boston Globe*[10,11] and others have printed numerous op-eds and editorials along the same lines long before the 'old grey lady' joined in.

Was it Ethical and Responsible to Offer Professional Opinions about Donald Trump without Having Personally Examined Him (*i.e.*, in violation of Goldwater)?

As many of the *Dangerous Case* authors wrote at the time, there was an abundance of evidence of Trump's character deficiencies publicly available to substantiate the conclusions we reached without the benefit of a professional examination (to which, any fair-minded observer would acknowledge, Mr. Trump, who considers himself "a very stable genius," would never agree to.)

For a variety of reasons which we have elaborated elsewhere,[12,13] we see the Goldwater Rule as anachronistic and a prejudicial "gag rule"[2] on members of the American Psychiatric Association, one that doesn't merit observance. Since 2017 it has been "honored in the breach" by numerous conscientious mental health professionals. [In 2018, our group, which included a significant number of internationally revered psychiatric leaders, formally proposed specific changes to the American Psychiatric Association to update Goldwater and bring it in line with advances in science and common sense. We never received a response.]

I think the extensive evidence of Donald Trump's actions and statements since 2017 by and large vindicate the validity of mental health professionals' assessments made seven years ago.

Was Our Writing Damaging to the Field, the Authors, or Patients Seeking Unbiased Professional Mental Health Care?

While our speaking out undoubtedly raised the profile of mental health professionals in the public's mind, it is harder to assess if, on balance, people view the professions more positively or not. I have certainly heard that some have seen our writings as "just what they'd expect" from highly educated elites; professionals who bear some of the stigma of their patients. Even some patients whose politics are more conservative, but who have managed to overcome their misgivings to enter treatment, still hesitate to acknowledge their political views during psychotherapy. They report fearing that the therapist (whose political views they assume tend to be liberal (and not unjustifiably) will hold their political views against them.

Others, of course, will feel supported in their personal assessment of Mr. Trump by seeing it validated in print by a variety of professionals.

I have no basis for assessing whether or how many patients may have not sought care because of fear of bias in the professionals. I have the general impression that dealing with mental health problems has become less stigmatized in recent times, but I have no way of connecting that to our writing.

When *The Dangerous Case* came out, there were plausible concerns that psychiatrists who spoke out in violation of Goldwater would face professional sanctions, *i.e.,* be reported to their state medical boards for ethical violations. To my knowledge this only happened once, and did not result in action against that psychiatrist's medical license.

Was it *Necessary* to Speak Out; *in other words* Did One Need to Be a Mental Health Professional to Recognize Trump was 'Off'?

On reflection this is the most fundamental question. We felt a "duty to warn," but was that grandiose, resting on the presumption that lay people couldn't discern what we mental health specialists saw? Or was it that our capability to describe and name the problem would add clarity and credibility to the general impression that Trump was psychologically disturbed? This begs the question of *diagnosis*: could we, should we have identified a specific diagnostic category that fit Trump to a T, and would that have served a bona fide purpose?

On this issue, our editor (B.L.) had urged the chapter authors of *the Dangerous Case* to refrain from specific diagnoses. Some elected to utilize DSM V diagnoses (narcissistic personality disorder, anti-social personality, malignant narcissism, bipolar disorder, dementia, etc.) as a way to educate the public on the spectrum of disorders in evidence. Others opined that the variations essentially represented "a distinction without a difference", given the consensus bottom line of Trump's psychological impairment.

Some other authors[14] declined to bring up diagnosis at all, not out of reverence for Goldwater, but because doing so would misdirect the focus. We emphasized that Donald Trump was *unfit* to serve in high office, and that asserting he had a diagnosable mental illness would only serve to offend and stigmatize.

Seven years on, there is general agreement about the central findings—Trump is unfit to serve as president. He is a self-obsessed, impulsive, vengeful, grandiose, compulsive liar who is unable to accept responsibility or acknowledge errors. Aside from those who are blinded by their near-religious devotion to him, *i.e.,* the MAGA followers, his psychological defects are universally recognizable. Whether the visibility of these aberrations was enhanced by some authors' use of diagnostic labels is arguable, but certainly at this point, outside of MAGA, a consensus assessment has formed, making further insistence on a specific diagnosis both superfluous and potentially counterproductive.

Conclusions

1) The central observations and cautions re. Donald Trump articulated by the gamut of mental health experts in *the Dangerous Case* have been validated by events of the past seven years. The book and similar writings by mental health workers raised awareness of the danger of Trump's psychological flaws.

2) Despite its violation of the ostensible ethical guard rails (the Goldwater Rule), the book served a bona fide public health interest.

3) It is unclear if the book and similar public utterances by mental health professionals damaged or enhanced the standing of the professions, or impacted the willingness of patients to seek mental health care.

The historic necessity of invoking a specific DSM V diagnosis to crystallize the public's understanding of the dangers inherent in Donald Trump as president remains debatable, but given the current state of public understanding, it appears no longer necessary. As Bandy Lee has pointed out (in our informal and occasional writing group composed of Bandy Lee, Ed Fisher, and me), seven years ago our mission was to illuminate those traits of Donald Trump that indicated a heightened risk of danger if he were in high office, not reach a diagnosis.

Leonard L. Glass, M.D., M.P.H. has served as an Associate Professor of Psychiatry (part-time) at Harvard Medical School, and taught at the Boston Psychiatric Society and Institute, Inc. for many years. He is an Attending Psychiatrist at McLean Hospital. He was acknowledged as a Distinguished Life Fellow of the American Psychiatric Association until he resigned in protest of the Goldwater Rule in 2017. He has written professionally about ethics, the psychology of men, and psychiatric risks of large groups. He has also educated the public on road rage, spectator violence at sporting events, and the dangerousness of Donald Trump.

References

The Dangerous Case of Donald Trump, Lee, B. ed St. Martin's Press, New York, 2017

Glass, L., https://www.bostonglobe.com/opinion/2017/07/28/let-psychiatrists-talk-about-trump-mental-state/hOBqRC8krC3AJBmrcAEEGM/story.html

Gourguechon, R., https://www.latimes.com/opinion/op-ed/la-oe-gourguechon-25th-amendment-leadership-mental-capacities-checklist-20170616-story.html

Brendel, R., https://www.psychiatrictimes.com/view/goldwater-rule-still-relevant, July 20, 2017,

Diagnosing from a Distance, Martin-Joy, J., Cambridge University Press, Cambridge, U.K., 2020

Glass, L., Should Psychiatrists Refrain from Commenting on Trump's Psychology, Lee, B, op.cit., p. 151-169.

https://en.wikipedia.org/wiki/Donald_Trump_Access_Hollywood_tape

https://www.nytimes.com/2018/01/10/opinion/is-mr-trump-nuts.html

https://www.nytimes.com/interactive/2024/07/11/opinion/editorials/donald-trump-2024-unfit.html

https://www.bostonglobe.com/opinion/2018/01/10/aren-diagnosing-trump-sounding-alarm/Kx995paa5Wv7Ns6UEOdErO/story.html

https://www.bostonglobe.com/opinion/2018/01/02/the-ethics-warning-public-about-dangerous-president/PimY2PNNKnOd1QG0lbc17N/story.html

https://www.statnews.com/2018/06/28/goldwater-rule-broken-psychiatrists/

https://www.statnews.com/2018/06/28/psychiatrists-goldwater-rule-rollback

Here I would acknowledge our informal and occasional writing group composed of Bandy Lee, Ed Fisher, and me.

https://bandyxlee.substack.com/p/seven-years-later-

PSYCHIATRIC ETHICS AND THE GOLDWATER RULE

Richard C. Friedman M.D. and Jennifer I. Downey M.D.

(This article was originally published in Psychodynamic Psychiatry, *46(3), 323-333. It is reprinted here with permission.)*

A recently published book edited by Bandy Lee of Yale University has provoked considerable controversy within organized psychiatry in the United States (Lee, 2017). In *The Dangerous Case of Donald Trump*, 27 psychiatrists and mental health professionals discuss Trump's psychology. The articles in *Dangerous Case* explore the potential dangerousness of President Donald Trump in light of his behavior. They also focus on the duties of psychiatrists as citizens and their responsibilities to their profession, especially when these duties and responsibilities appear to be in conflict. The reasons for the conflict are demonstrated by the prescriptions and restrictions of the Goldwater rule on the conduct of psychiatrists.

ETHICS AND THE GOLDWATER RULE

Before going on, let us say that the so-called "Goldwater rule" does not really exist as such. The wording forbidding certain behavior by psychiatrists is found in an APA Annotation to the AMA Ethics Code first made in 1973 as follows:

On occasion psychiatrists are asked for an opinion about an individual who is in the light of public attention or who has disclosed information about himself/herself through public media. In such circumstances, a psychiatrist may share with the public his or her expertise about psychiatric issues in general. However, it is unethical for a psychiatrist to offer a professional opinion unless he or she has conducted an examination and has been granted proper authorization for such a statement (American Psychiatric Association, 2009).

In March of 2017, shortly after Donald Trump's presidential inauguration, having let the wording about the Goldwater rule stand since 1973, the American Psychiatric Association (APA) felt it necessary to further explain this advice, writing:

A diagnosis is not required for an opinion to be professional. Instead, when a psychiatrist renders an opinion about the affect, behavior, speech, or other presentation of an individual that draws on the skills, training, expertise, and/or knowledge inherent in the practice of psychiatry, the opinion is a professional one (American Psychiatric Association, 2017).

There has been debate about whether these additional comments broadened the way the Goldwater rule was originally formulated. The official position of the APA is that the few sentences added in 2017 did not change the meaning of the Goldwater rule. According to this view, explication is not revision. Critics of the APA's position commented that the APA seemed to be discouraging open, honest discussion of the issues by psychiatrists (Lee, 2017, Sandberg, 2018).

INTERVIEW WITH BANDY LEE, M.D.

Recently, Dr. Bandy Lee agreed to be interviewed about *The Dangerous Case of Donald Trump*. We publish this interview in this issue of *Psychodynamic Psychiatry* (Sandberg, 2018, 46(3) 323–334). We (Friedman and Downey) are grateful to Larry Sandberg, M.D., a psychiatrist and psychoanalyst on the faculty of Columbia University Department of Psychiatry, for interviewing Dr. Lee. Our editorial does not review Dr. Lee's book; however, we do comment on its quality. In our view, *The Dangerous Case of Donald Trump* is thought-provoking and, although provocative, falls within acceptable professional bounds. In reaching this conclusion we agree with Claire Pouncey's comments in *The New England Journal of Medicine* on February 1, 2018. Pouncey wrote:

I expect that the APA will denounce and dismiss this book and its authors, but I encourage others not to do so.... I believe that the APA...should take caution not to enforce an annotation that undermines the overriding public health and safety mandate that applies to all physicians. Standards of professional ethics and professionalism change with time and circumstance, and psychiatry's reaction to one misstep in 1964 should not entail another in 2017 (p. 407).

The overall purpose of Lee's volume appeared to be to bear witness to Trump's potentially dangerous behavior, which threatens the safety and security of the general public, and to direct attention to four major domains: (1) Trump's mental health versus possible mental illness; (2) Trump's behavior, whether it is moral or immoral; (3) the social appropriateness or inappropriateness of the public behavior of political figures (in this case Trump); and (4) most importantly, the right of psychiatrists to engage in political advocacy versus the requirement that they remain politically passive.

The contributors were concerned about Donald Trump's behavior to the point of being alarmed about its effect on the state. They saw it as their responsibility to rapidly transmit this concern and alarm to the general public. This stimulated an underlying question: Exactly who should decide what is transmitted to the general public about issues such as the ones outlined? Should educational efforts be relegated to the APA, for example? In fact, should the APA, whether formally or informally, somehow "regulate" discussion of the issues?

FACT Magazine, THE GOLDWATER RULE, AND PSYCHOANALYTIC PSYCHOLOGY

The Goldwater rule was adopted by the APA in 1973 in reaction to a now infamous questionnaire published in 1964 by *FACT Magazine*, which polled psychiatrists for their opinion on the mental health of Barry Goldwater, the Republican candidate for president (Boroson, 1964).

The psychological model used to understand and treat patients in the 1960's and 1970's was strongly influenced by psychoanalytic psychology. In fact, there was basically no other developmental model than the psychoanalytic one that psychiatrists could apply to the clinical problems they faced daily. The historical issues involving psychiatric models of the mind as they changed in the late 1970's and early 1980's are especially relevant for understanding psychodynamic psychiatry today.

In the 1970's, many psychiatrists were as amused as the general public by the aspects of psychoanalysis that were satirized in novels, cartoons, and films. Everyone, everywhere, seemed to have an openly expressed Oedipus complex, and satirists found easy targets in which all men wished to sleep with their mothers. Not only did women seem to passionately desire their fathers, they all seemed to envy men for having a phallus! Subsequent political-psychological developments have demonstrated that the male phallus seems to have retained its symbolic weight in American politics.

In our view, most psychiatrists today do not speak openly about people they have not directly examined. In the 1960's, most psychiatrists did not openly speculate about Barry Goldwater's psychology in response to the *FACT Magazine* questionnaire—but some did. An outraged public and alarmed professional community influenced the APA to include a Goldwater rule in its statements of ethics (Pouncey, 2018). This decision probably has acted as a brake on psychiatrists who might otherwise have been tempted to be reckless in their speculations about public figures.

Meanwhile, at the same time as the Goldwater rule was adopted by the APA, the very broad and often nonspecific psychoanalytic developmental model of the mind that psychiatry was using was in the process of being challenged and then replaced by the descriptive model of the *DSM-III* (Bayer, 1981).

The *DSM-III* marked a radical change in the way behavior was viewed by psychiatrists, and seemed to many (ourselves included) to be a useful and helpful move in the right direction. It added a measure of specificity to the behavioral model associated with a circumscribed perspective that limited speculation about human motivation.

It is difficult to express how *powerful* the impact was of the adoption of a criteria-based diagnostic approach for looking at psychology, psychopathology, and psychological development.

PSYCHOANALYTIC MODEL OF THE MIND VERSUS THE *DSM-III*

The psychoanalytic model of the mind that dominated psychiatry prior to the *DSM-III* was broad, even global. It tended to encourage those who wished to make speculations about the entire range of human experience and behavior. The descriptive, symptom-based model that psychiatry uses today cannot be applied in such a fashion.

Modern psychiatry has its hands full focusing on psychiatric disorders rather than the entire range of human experience and behavior.

TIMES CHANGE

Times change and today different issues are of immediate concern. This pertains to the public presentation of the self by psychiatrists. When the psychoanalytic model of the mind was in ascendency, there was a general sense that psychoanalytically oriented psychiatrists should not be openly political.

It was widely believed that an appropriate professional role for psychoanalysts and psychiatrists was to be more or less neutral in public situations. To be openly expressive might inhibit the formation of transference by patients in psychoanalytically oriented therapies. In other words, the concern was that open political advocacy might have negative effects on the *psychoanalytic treatment itself*. There was no evidence supporting this, but nonetheless, it was believed by many psychoanalysts (Schachter, 2002).

We believe the attitudes and values adopted by a professional culture during its formative years can have a lasting influence. Attitudes and values of the past may still influence many psychoanalysts and contemporary psychodynamic psychiatrists to be cautious in their presentation of self, particularly with respect to political advocacy.

When is a psychiatrist not a psychiatrist — can they have a personal opinion ??

PSYCHIATRIC OPINION ABOUT PUBLIC FIGURES

The term "professional opinion," according to the APA, should be understood as follows:

> …when a psychiatrist renders an opinion about the affect, behavior, speech, or other presentation of an individual that draws on the skills, training, expertise, and/or knowledge inherent in the practice of psychiatry, the opinion is a professional one (APA, 2018).

The Ethics Committee of the APA has clarified that the rule applies to all professional opinions offered by psychiatrists, not just diagnoses. For example, saying an individual does not have a mental disorder would also constitute a professional opinion. These few sentences of explication/clarification of the original Goldwater rule that the Ethics Committee of the American Psychiatric Association added in 2017 are confusing, and seem to extend its meaning in ways that are impossible to implement.

Once individuals have completed psychiatric residency, their opinions about *everyone* draw on skills, training, expertise, and knowledge inherent in the practice of psychiatry. This applies to opinions about parents, children, siblings, wives, husbands, lovers, friends, professional colleagues, and public celebrities.

In fact, most life experience is influenced by one's psychiatric knowledge and training once one becomes a psychiatrist. There is no way to edit this perspective out, which may or may not have an inhibiting effect on critical thought depending on context. With respect to inhibition, a quotation from Ring Lardner (1920) comes to mind. "Are you lost, Daddy?" I asked tenderly. "*Shut up*," he explained.

This may, in part, be why some people experienced the 2017 explication as provocative. It seemed to demand, "Don't say *anything*." In discussing this issue informally with colleagues, we discovered that many are puzzled about what led the American Psychiatric Association to add these sentences to the Goldwater rule in 2017.

LYING

Donald Trump was a celebrity before he became president, and his celebrity status has now been greatly amplified. The public image of his self appears contradictory, seemingly expressing a paradoxical idea, "I lie, but trust me anyway."

The conflation of lying with the demand for unconditional trust is a direct challenge to the common-sense experience of social relationships that most of us rely on. While not directly stating this verbally, Trump's behavior can be taken to mean, "Trust me because of who I am and disregard what I say,"—which challenges the commonly accepted American assumption that the electorate should be openly informed.

As psychiatrists, we are aware of the influence of celebrities on the psychological development of children and adolescents. Will young people get an unspoken message that they can aspire to be president someday and can lie to achieve this goal? Thinking like this involves mobilizing our identities as psychiatrists and comments on the character traits displayed by the public personality who appears on display day after day.

Is it possible to think about the meaning of all this without utilizing some of the knowledge and values of our psychiatric education? We don't think so.

Allen Frances, M.D., has condemned Trump's behavior, but has pointedly commented that organized psychiatry cannot rescue the United States from the fact that our democracy has made its decision and he is a duly elected president. This view holds aside the troubling issue that Russia, our age-old adversary, may have had its thumb on the voting scale. Frances has emphasized that millions of people voted for Trump and that psychiatry, by labeling him mentally unbalanced in some sense or other, should not be placed in the situation of attempting to save our democracy from itself (Wilson, 2017).

The citizens who voted for Trump did so knowingly. He had been a public figure long before he ran for president, and many of the behaviors mentioned have long been on public view.

THE PRESIDENT'S SOCIAL ROLE

Rulers of great nations and empires tend to have historically prescribed and ritualized social roles. Think of a scene from the Netflix drama, *The Crown*, in which Churchill dispenses advice to the king. Churchill tells him to show as little of his private self to the general public as possible. He explains that the general public wishes to see the kingly/queenly *role* enacted. and this role serves the Commonwealth well. This scene captures the idea that the social roles of "King" and "Queen" have been historically established by precedent and tradition. Public display of the king or queen in this role, which emphasizes duty, formality, and ritual, connects the past to the present and strengthens the identity of subjects throughout the British Empire.

American presidents have done this to some extent as well. Donald Trump does sometimes adjust his behavior to historically determined expectations, for instance, when presiding over state dinners. However, Trump often insists on public acceptance of aspects of his "private" self. Whether an actual self or a fictional creation, the character called "Trump" frequently uses the presidential platform to be unmannerly or even distasteful to others.

As a psychiatrist, one wonders what type of behavior might emerge next. As citizens we can't help but notice that one function of Trump's public presentation of self is to create an image distinct and separate from all previous images associated with a presidential role. The image—if generally endorsed—would change the meaning of what it means to "be presidential." The voters have the right to determine this, of course. As professional psychiatrists, we cannot help but consider such questions such as (1) the effect on groups of charismatic leaders, (2) the psychological mechanisms by which groups become mobs, and (3) the psychological mechanisms involving scapegoating and persecuting others.

Below, we comment on one of Trump's specific types of abuse of others where we see a clear ethical issue, and where we do believe the profession of psychiatry has a particular responsibility—as a profession—to object to.

MOCKERY OF THE DISABLED

Donald Trump's infamous mockery of a physically disabled reporter is now part of history. It happened in November 2015, at the Myrtle Beach Convention Center when Trump hoisted a hand up, flailed his arms, and imitated a New York Tim*es* reporter who has a condition called arthrogryposis. Although Trump denied this event, it was caught on videotape, and the mockery was later confirmed by the *Los Angeles Times* and the *Washington Post,* among others (Spayd, 2017).

Many individuals have objected to this behavior, but we have failed to find a single organization of physicians that has done so. We suggest that it is not only appropriate but ethically mandated for physicians, whether individually or in groups, to condemn abuse of the disabled. And for psychiatrists—how far is mockery of the physically disabled from mockery of the psychologically disabled? As physicians, we are responsible for speaking out against abuse of all disabled people.

DENIAL AND POLITICAL ADVOCACY BY PROFESSIONAL ASSOCIATIONS

Some of the contributors to *Dangerous Case* observed that denial and political passivity on the part of the general public and professional organizations has been skillfully exploited by charismatic dictators of the past (Lifton, 2017). This point has been emphasized by political historians as well, especially in discussing the history of fascism in years gone by (Albright, 2018). This denial often led to political apathy and minimization of the significance of events that history has shown to be real and present dangers to democracies.

CONCLUSION

Dangerous Case calls attention not only to Donald Trump's behavior but also to that of the psychiatric profession itself. What is the appropriate balance between an individual psychiatrist's duties and psychiatric identity and a citizen's duties and identity (Dodes & Schachter, 2017)? Clearly the present political situation in the United States is one in which psychiatric identity and responsibility, as currently defined by the American Psychiatric Association, can conflict with civic identity and duty. The APA's addition of the few sentences to the Goldwater rule in 2017 were meant to clarify and explain aspects of the Goldwater rule. In our view, they exacerbated the conflict between professional and civic rights and responsibilities.

One reason that *Dangerous Case* aroused opposition in some quarters may have been that it seemed to reach out to the general public almost as a hypothetical "committee of the whole" and apparently to de-emphasize, if not bypass, more nuanced, differentiated channels of communication between the psychiatric and non-psychiatric communities. Of course, a reason for taking this route could be—as some have argued—that the power of the president is so great, especially but not exclusively with regard to risk of nuclear war, that the contributors felt a responsibility as citizens to have their voices heard rapidly by the public.

The trading of insults by the dictator of North Korea—so called "Rocket man"—and Trump exacerbated anxiety throughout the world. This anxiety was amplified by the leaders' public posturing about whose nuclear button was bigger (@CNNPolitics, 2018).

We add our voices to the many others who have commented on Trump's dangerous behavior. We believe that the populace should be continually educated about the behavior of our leaders, as a matter of civic responsibility. Although the American Psychiatric Association does have the inherent status to be the voice of American Psychiatry, nonetheless it must be wary of attempting to regulate the open expression of ideas by psychiatrists or (inadvertently) acting to censor discussion of controversial matters.

Professional associations including the American Psychiatric Association serve scientific–clinical functions but also guild–political functions. We have the highest regard for the APA's Committee on Ethics, but well-informed people can have principled disagreements without personal conflict. The contributors to *Dangerous Case* emphasize that we live in unusual and unusually dangerous times. Never before has an American with a similar behavioral profile as Donald Trump occupied the office of Chief Executive and Commander-in-Chief. Many discussants and critics have listed the physical and mental defects and disabilities of former presidents and observed that the government functioned nonetheless. Trump's behavioral profile is unique among all American presidents, and the authors of Lee's volume argue that he is uniquely dangerous and the public needs to be warned.

As we have stated earlier, we are not critically assessing Lee's volume, chapter by chapter. We do conclude, however, that its perspective is sobering and worthy of respect. We endorse the need for widespread, open discussion of the President's behavior, including by physicians, whose concern for public health and safety is mandated by our profession (Pouncey, 2018). Psychiatrists cannot abrogate their civic responsibilities because of their professional identities and social roles.

Richard C. Friedman, M.D., had been Editor of the peer-reviewed journal, Psychodynamic Psychiatry, for eight years at the time of his death in 2020. At that time, he was Clinical Professor of Psychiatry at Weill-Cornell School of Medicine and Lecturer in Psychiatry at Columbia University College of Physicians and Surgeons. His work on sexual orientation and identity in both men and women with Dr. Jennifer Downey spanned over twenty years. A leader of thought in psychiatry, Dr. Friedman was willing to assess psychoanalytic theory critically and test it against biological psychiatry, neuroscience, and research psychology. Psychodynamic Psychiatry embodies his beliefs.

Jennifer Downey, M.D., is Clinical Professor of Psychiatry at the Columbia University College of Physicians and Surgeons and Faculty Member at the Columbia University Center for Psychoanalytic Training and Research. She and Dr. Cesar Alfonso serve as joint Editors-in-Chief of Psychodynamic Psychiatry. She and Dr. Richard Friedman co-authored Sexual Orientation and Psychodynamic Psychotherapy: Sexual Science and Clinical Practice *(Columbia University Press, 2008). They published 24 peer-reviewed articles together between 1993 and 2016. Dr. Downey is a psychodynamic psychiatrist whose areas of interest are women's health, sexual minorities and issues of sexual identity, and teaching psychodynamic interventions to medical clinicians.*

References

Albright, M. (2018). *Fascism: A warning*. New York, NY: Harper Collins.

American Psychiatric Association. (2009). *The principles of medical ethics with annotations especially applicable to psychiatry* (Rev. ed.). Washington, DC: Author.

American Psychiatric Association. (1980). *The diagnostic and statistical manual of mental disorders* (3rd ed.). Washington, DC: American Psychiatric Association Press.

American Psychiatric Association. (2017, March 15). APA remains committed to supporting Goldwater Rule. Retrieved from https://www.psychiatry.org/ newsroom/apa-blogs/apa-blog/2017/03/apa-remains-committed-to-supporting-goldwater-rule

American Psychiatric Association. (2018, January 9). Calls for end to "armchair" psychiatry. Retrieved from https://www.psychiatry.org/newsroom/newsreleases/apa-calls-for-end-to-armchair-psychiatry

Associated Press. (2018, March 18). Trump savages the FBI, accuses Comey of lying under oath—Cites Fox. Retrieved from https://www.haaretz.com/us-news

Bayer, R. V. (1981). *Homosexuality and american psychiatry: The politics of diagnosis*. New York, NY: Basic Books.

Boroson, W. (1964). What psychiatrists say about Goldwater: 1189 psychiatrists say Goldwater is psychologically unfit to be president. *FACT Magazine, 1*(5), 2464.

@CNNPolitics. (2018, January 3). Trump tweets about nuclear war with North Korea. Retrieved from https://www.cnn.com/2018/01/02/politics/...trump-northkorea-nuclear/index.html

Dodes, L., & Schachter, J. (2017, Feb. 13). Letter to the Editor: Mental health professionals warn about Trump. *The New York Times*. Retrieved from https:// www.nytimes.com/2017/02/13/opinion/mental-health-professionalswarn-about-trump.html

Friedman, R. C. (1988). *Male homosexuality: A contemporary psychoanalytic perspective*. New Haven, CT: Yale University Press.

Friedman, R. C., & Downey, J. I. (2008). *Sexual orientation and psychodynamic psychotherapy: Sexual science and clinical practice*. New York, NY: Columbia University Press.

Goldman-Rakic, P. (1995). Architecture of the pre-frontal cortex and the central executive function. *Annals of the New York Academy of Sciences, 769*(1), 71-84.

Gonzales, G., & Henning-Smith, C. (2017). Health disparities by sexual orientation: Results and implications from the behavioral-risk factor surveillance system. *Journal of Community Health, 420*(6), 1163-1172.

Lardner, R. (1920). *The young immigrunts.* Indianapolis IN: Bobbs-Merrill.

Lee, B. X. (Ed.). (2017). *The dangerous case of Donald Trump: 27 psychiatrists and mental health experts assess a president.* New York, NY: St. Martin's Press.

Lifton, R. J. (2017). Our witness to malignant normality. In B. X. Lee (Ed.), *The dangerous case of Donald Trump: 27 psychiatrists and mental health experts assess a president* (pp. xv-xix). New York, NY: St. Martin Press.

Pouncey, C. (2018). President Trump's mental health—Is it morally permissible to comment? *New England Journal of Medicine, 378*(5), 405-407.

Raifman, J., Moscoe, S., Austin, B., Hatzenbuehler, M. L., & Galea, S. (2018). Association of state laws permitting denial of services to same-sex couples with mental distress in sexual minority adults: A difference-in-difference-in-differences analysis. *JAMA Psychiatry.* [Advanced online publication]. Retrieved from https://doi.org/10.1001/jamapsychiatry.2018.0757

Sandberg, L. S. (2018). Interview with Bandy Lee. *Psychodynamic Psychiatry, 46*(3), 335-355.

Schachter, J. (2002). *Transference: Shibboleth or albatross.* Hillsdale, NJ: Analytic.

Spayd, L. (2017, January 10). Not "she said, he said": Mockery, plain and simple. Public Editor. *The New York Times.* Retrieved from https://www.nytimes.com/2017/01/10/public-editor/trump-streep-golden-globes.html

Wilson, F. P. (2017, November 20). Misdiagnosing Trump: Doc-to-doc with Allen Frances, MD. *Medpage Today.* Retrieved from https://www.medpagetoday.com/psychiatry/generalpsychiatry/67728

A RE-EXAMINATION OF THE GOLDWATER RULE

JERROLD M. POST, M.D., AND BANDY X. LEE, M.D., M.DIV.

(This essay was coauthored in 2019 for the Psychiatric Times *but was not accepted; here it is slightly abbreviated, and Dr. Lee's additional comments kept in brackets.)*

The 2016 presidential campaign and his presidency led to an extraordinary outpouring concerning Donald J. Trump as delusional, crazy, psychopathic, narcissistic, manic-depressive, and mentally disturbed. But few psychiatrists were offering opinions about the clinical psychology of the Republican candidate. Why not? The answer could be found in the title of this article, the Goldwater rule, which refers to Section 7 of the code of medical ethics particularly applicable to psychiatrists, the last prong of which is:

> On occasion psychiatrists are asked for an opinion about an individual who is in the light of public attention, or who has disclosed information about himself/herself through public media. It is unethical for a psychiatrist to offer a professional opinion unless he/she has conducted an examination and has been granted proper authorization for such a statement.

Because of the outpouring of psychiatric diagnoses by non-clinicians referred to above, the leadership of the American Psychiatric Association (APA) saw fit in the fall of 2016 to post on its website a warning to its members:

> The unique atmosphere of this year's election cycle may lead some to want to psychoanalyze the candidates, but to do so would not only be

unethical, it would be irresponsible.

This article questions the absolute manner in which the ethical prohibition is applied. It argues that there are some unusual circumstances where psychiatrists may ethically contribute, indeed are ethically obliged to contribute to the discourse concerning the mental stability or dangerous traits of the subject of concern, as long as a diagnosis is not proffered.

University of Minnesota psychiatrist Dr. Jerome Kroll, who has recommended calling for termination of the Goldwater rule, has stated:

> I am a citizen. If I have something to say, what I say might be stupid. What I say may embarrass psychiatry, but it's certainly not medically unethical. I think [Donald Trump] comes as close to the narcissistic description as one would find. I think that would disqualify him. I am breaking the Goldwater rule as we speak.

Indeed, these words are reminiscent of those of Dr. Alan Stone, Professor of Psychiatry and the Law at Harvard, when he participated in a plenary symposium Dr. Post organized for an American Psychiatric Association (APA) annual meeting some 15 years ago on the ethical dilemmas of the Goldwater rule. After recalling proudly that he was the only member of the board who voted against the Goldwater rule's adoption when it was proposed in 1973, he stated, "You cannot legislate against stupidity. It is not unethical to be stupid." He then walked to the front of the stage, where the entire ethics committee was sitting in the front row. Dr. Stone then said, "I would like to confess in front of the ethics committee that I have violated the Goldwater rule I believe eight times." Then crossing his hands, as if in handcuffs, he said, "So, arrest me."

[Nevertheless, in 2018, Dr. Stone denounced Dr. Lee in a *Lawfare* article entitled, "The psychiatrist's Goldwater rule in the Trump era," stating:

> Dr. Lee, author and editor of *The Dangerous Case of Donald Trump: 27 Psychiatrists and Mental Health Experts Assess a President* ... believes that Trump's mental disabilities were (and presumably are) so severe and the risks accompanying the powers of the presidency so great that she had an overriding "duty to warn." But there is no such explicit obligation in the medical or psychiatric canons of ethics.... The publication of this

book obviously defies the Goldwater rule—which, moreover, has been strengthened by the American Psychiatric Association in the Trump era. It had been widely understood in its original formulation as forbidding a diagnosis. The new formulation, however, might be read to forbid any comment framed in professional psychiatric terms and expertise in a political or electoral context (Stone, 2018).

It defied understanding for Dr. Lee how Dr. Stone would so radically change his position with the arrival of Donald Trump, such that Dr. Stone would not even see that the very expansion of the Goldwater rule upon Trump's inauguration was a political act, since nothing in psychiatric scholarship or practice had changed. Yet, he was not an exception; many such inexplicable inconsistencies would arise with the Goldwater rule in the Trump era.]

The Goldwater rule

The Goldwater rule refers to Section 7 of the "Principles of Medical Ethics, With Annotations Especially Applicable to Psychiatry," i.e., the American Psychiatric Association Code of Ethics. This ethical principle is a masterpiece of internal contradiction. On the one hand:

"A physician shall recognize a responsibility to participate in activities contributing to an improved community" and "Psychiatrists are encouraged to serve society" and "may interpret and share with the public their expertise in the various psychosocial issues that may affect mental health and illness."

Yet, on the other hand:

On occasion psychiatrists are asked for an opinion about an individual who is in the light of public attention, or who has disclosed information about himself/herself through public media. It is unethical for a psychiatrist to offer a professional opinion unless he/she has conducted an examination and has been granted proper authorization for such a statement.

For Dr. Post, the dilemma was no more dramatically and absurdly evidenced than during the Persian Gulf crisis of 1990–91. On the basis of a political personality profile that he developed of Saddam Hussein from his base at the George Washington University, one that was widely featured in print and electronic media, in late 1990, he was invited to testify before two congressional committees holding hearings on the Gulf Crisis: Les Aspin's House Armed Services Committee and Lee Hamilton's House Foreign Affairs Committee. Saddam Hussein had been widely characterized as "the madman of the Middle East," and there was considerable perplexity concerning what made him tick.

Policies were being developed that, in Dr. Post's judgment, were insufficiently informed by an accurate picture of Saddam Hussein's political psychology. This was an extraordinary opportunity for a political psychologist to present the principal conclusions of Hussein's profile to legislators charged with the responsibility for the policy development process, and to contribute to their understanding of the complex cultural, historical, political, and psychological influences on Saddam Hussein's decision making. After this testimony was presented, in a public forum Ambassador Sam Lewis, then president of the U.S. Institute of Peace, cited the profile as a "contribution of the highest order to the national welfare." The testimony was cited by several congressmen as having contributed to their decision-making during the crisis.

Then, the chair of the APA's Council of Psychiatry and International Affairs, on which Dr. Post served, called, and Dr. Post was anticipating a compliment for his contribution to American psychiatry. Instead, he heard, "Jerry, the APA has received letters about your profile of Saddam, and there is reason to believe you may have violated the Canons of Ethics of the American Psychiatric Association."

Apparently, an article about personality profiling, drawing on his Saddam Hussein profile, had appeared in the "Science News" section of the *New York Times*. This led to complaints that he had violated Section 7 of the Canons of Ethics of the APA because he had presented publicly a professional opinion about Hussein without interviewing him and without his authorization. Dr. Post nearly exploded: "Have you read the profile?"

"Well, no," the chair acknowledged.

"Then perhaps you should before rendering such judgments. The profile is not a psychiatric expert opinion." Dr. Post added, "I think there is a duty to warn, involving a kind of Tarasoff principle, for the assessments of Saddam's political personality and leadership that are guiding policy seem to me to be off—he had been widely characterized as "the madman of the Middle East"—and policy decisions are being made based on errant perceptions, which could lead to significant loss of life….

"Accordingly," Dr. Post concluded, "it would have been unethical to have withheld this assessment. I believed I had a duty to warn."

Dr. Post faxed the profile to him and heard no more on the matter, but the conversation continued to trouble him. How can it be that a presentation deemed to be "a contribution of the highest order to the national welfare" could simultaneously raise questions concerning an ethical violation? Other academic specialists from the ranks of psychology, political science, and history regularly contribute to public discourse on political figures without having interviewed the subject, but for psychiatrists to do so is considered an ethical violation. The ethical principle seemed extreme and overdrawn.

First, diagnostic methods have dramatically changed since 1964. In 1973, when the Goldwater rule entered the books, it was already considered outdated. Dr. Post was by that time developing pilot programs within the Central Intelligence Agency (CIA) to produce political-psychological profiles to provide assistance to U.S. government foreign policy officials conducting summit meetings and other high-level negotiations with foreign leaders, to assist in dealing with political-military crises, based on which he founded the CIA Center for the Analysis of Personality and Political Behavior. Since 1980, objective observations of behavior came to be valued over introspective interviews, and the rise of forensic psychiatry placed an increasing emphasis on functional assessments, such as evaluations of fitness or dangerousness, in which personal interviews and consent are less relevant.

In the course of examining the use and potential for abuse of psychiatric profiles, the APA Psychohistory Task Force carefully considered the use of profiles in support of national security. The report made an exception for psychiatric profiles that were prepared for the use of the government, not only indicating that they were not considered unethical, but also singling them out as positively contributing to the national welfare. The task force determined that profiles of significant international figures could be helpful—and were in fact necessary in some cases—to support the national interest. They made positive reference to the profile, *The Mind of Adolf Hitler*, prepared during World War II by psychoanalyst Walter Langer at the request of Bill Donovan, the director of the Office of Strategic Services, the predecessor organization to the CIA (Post, 1993).

This judgment was of great comfort to Dr. Post in his national security role, but provided no comfort when he assumed his position as director of the Political Psychology Program at the Elliott School of International Affairs at the George Washington University. There, part of his role was to contribute to the national dialogue from the perspective of political psychology, as exemplified by his testimony concerning Saddam Hussein. Thus, on several occasions when he believed he had something useful to contribute, he did not, constrained by the ethical canon.

One such occasion, which he continued to regret, was the Federal Bureau of Investigation (FBI) siege of the Branch Davidian compound in Waco, Texas, in 1993. Based on a profile of David Koresh by an FBI consulting psychologist, who had judged Koresh to be a psychopath, the FBI employed a strategy of increasing escalation of pressure, with sound bombardment and flashing lights going around the clock. Dr. Post had been following Koresh for several years, and he had come to see him, like many charismatic cult leaders, as a narcissistic borderline. Dr. Post was concerned that these FBI tactics could drive him "over the border" and lead him to seek martyrdom. Sam Donaldson on ABC's Prime Time Live interviewed Dr. Post and, although Dr. Post expressed concern about the possibly counterproductive effects of the FBI tactics, he did not provide his at-a-distance personality profile assessment of Koresh, which would have given substance to his concerns.

Troubled by the constraints posed by overly broad ethical guidance, Dr. Post sought an audience with the APA ethics committee. Although they reassured him that they considered his contributions to be positive and not ethical violations, they suggested that he formally seek guidance from the committee in terms of submitting a question. Hence, in 2008, Dr. Post submitted the following question:

> Does the ethical prohibition embodied in Section 7, Paragraph 3 of the Annotations apply to psychologically informed leadership studies based on careful research that do not specify a clinical diagnosis and are designed to enhance public and governmental understanding?

This is the response:

> The psychological profiling of historical figures designed to enhance public and governmental understanding of these individuals does not conflict with the ethical principles outlined in Section 7, Paragraph 3, as long as the psychological profiling does not include a clinical diagnosis and is that of scholarly research that has been subject to peer review and academic

scrutiny, and is based on relevant standards of scholarship.

With the amendment to the principles in the question and answer from the ethics committee quoted above, Dr. Post deemed the constraints upon psychiatrists contributing to public awareness of leaders of concern considerably loosened. This led to his publishing, *Narcissism and Politics: Dreams of Glory* (Post, 2015).

In early 2018, however, the APA seemed to reverse its stance once again. Not only had it expanded the Goldwater rule shortly after Donald Trump's inauguration—to prohibit not just diagnosis but all commentary—it even exceeded its jurisdiction. Dr. Lee had resigned from APA membership in 2007, objecting to its receiving a third of its revenue from pharmaceutical companies, and she did not consider herself subject to its guild rules when she published *The Dangerous Case of Donald Trump*, which became an instant *New York Times* bestseller, and within months raised the issue of the president's mental fitness to the number one topic of national conversation. Alarmingly for her, the APA publicly accused her and her renowned colleagues of "armchair psychiatry" and "using psychiatry for political or self-aggrandizing purposes," which seemed to her not only incorrect, but the very violation of its expanded Goldwater rule it was accusing them of committing (it had not evaluated Dr. Lee nor obtained consent to speak about her as a public figure; additionally, ethics violations were supposed to be investigated confidentially, and the results not revealed until a conclusion is reached). Drs. Judith Herman and Robert Jay Lifton, both Distinguished Life Fellows of the APA, supported Dr. Lee in writing a letter to the APA leadership:

Dear Drs. Everett, Stewart, and Griffith:

We, authors of *The Dangerous Case of Donald Trump*, on behalf of hundreds of colleagues who have joined [us], write to respond to the American Psychiatric Association, which recently (January 9, 2018), called for an end to "armchair psychiatry" and using psychiatry for "political or self-aggrandizing purposes." We agree....

Where we disagree with the APA is in the recent expansion (March 16, 2017) of the "Goldwater Rule" to prohibit any form of commentary on public figures. Such commentary is both appropriate and necessary when it pertains to political leaders responsible for public safety. When a man who has the authority to initiate a nuclear strike shows signs of mental instability, we believe that our profession fails in our ethical duty if we

185

remain silent.

> We have written our book to help educate and warn the public, on the basis of our professional judgment, of the danger we face. We have agreed to take no personal royalties from the book, and we have no conflicts of interest.

> We call on the APA to reconsider its recent ill-conceived expansion of the "Goldwater Rule." We seek further exchange on these issues with our colleagues in the APA, issues that go to the heart of our professional responsibilities.

> B.X.L., J.L.H., and R.J.L.

None of the letter's addressees, but the Trustees of the APA responded as a whole, stating merely that a "robust discussion" on the Goldwater rule had already been had within the APA, and therefore the matter was closed.

[This was around the time when Dr. Post contacted Dr. Lee, and they began their weekly discussions on how to speak about the then-president in a way that did not violate their conscience and their sense of ethics, which lasted almost two years. Dr. Post invited Dr. Lee to join his group of political psychologists, but Dr. Lee maintained that her background as a social psychiatrist, or as any psychiatrist, obligated her to the preamble of their medical ethics code (which the APA adopted), which states: "a physician must recognize responsibility to patients … as well as to society" (American Medical Association, 2001). Dr. Lee believed that they had a "duty to warn," not just as an extension of the Tarasoff doctrine (the duty to protect a non-patient from danger) but as a duty to protect society as a primary obligation (society was their "patient"). Dr. Lee felt most ingratiated when Dr. Post contributed to the second edition of *The Dangerous Case of Donald Trump* and told Dr. Lee that he was echoing her language when he used the word, "dangerous", in his highly-prescient and discerning book, *Dangerous Charisma: The Political Psychology of Donald Trump and His Followers* (Post, 2019). She witnessed Dr. Post be betrayed when an APA president-elect promised to allow him to chair a commission to reexamine the Goldwater rule, which gave him immense hope, only to cease contact with him once in office. Dr. Post waited, truly to the end of his life, to have the opportunity to chair such a commission. And he would die from Covid-19, grossly mismanaged by the very dangerous leader he tried to warn against. Because of his career in political personality profiling, Dr. Post continued to receive media requests but was besieged with misgivings because of the APA's stance on the Goldwater rule. He stated, "I am increasingly uncomfortable in not having commented upon the psychiatric diagnoses offered by people without psychiatrist training and experience. It feels to me unethical to not have contributed at this perilous time." Yet, Dr. Lee would assert that he contributed more than anyone.]

Jerrold M. Post, M.D., was Professor of Psychiatry, Political Psychology, and International Affairs and Director of the Political Psychology Program at George Washington University. Dr. Post had a twenty-one-year career with the Central Intelligence Agency, where he founded and directed the Center for the Analysis of Personality and Political Behavior. He is the recipient of numerous awards and author of numerous, highly-acclaimed works in political psychology. After the invasion of Kuwait, Dr. Post's profile of Saddam Hussein was featured prominently in the media. His last book was, Dangerous Charisma: The Political Psychology of Donald Trump and His Followers.

Bandy X. Lee, M.D., M.Div., is a forensic and social psychiatrist who taught at Yale School of Medicine and Yale Law School for 17 years before joining the Harvard Program in Psychiatry and the Law. She edited The Dangerous Case of Donald Trump: 27 Psychiatrists and Mental Health Experts Assess a President, *in order to warn the public of a national public health emergency. She is President of the World Mental Health Coalition and Cofounder of the Violence Prevention Institute. She most recently authored* The Psychology of Trump Contagion: An Existential Danger to American Democracy and All Humankind.

References

American Medical Association (2001). *AMA principles of medical ethics.* Chicago, IL: American Medical Association. Retrieved from https://code-medical-ethics. ama-assn.org/principles

American Psychiatric Association (2013). *The principles of medical ethics with annota-*

tions especially applicable to psychiatry. Arlington, VA: American Psychiatric Association. Retrieved from https://www.psychiatry.org/psychiatrists/practice/ethics

American Psychiatric Association (2018). *APA calls for end to "armchair psychiatry".* Washington, DC: American Psychiatric Association. Retrieved from https://www.psychiatry.org/news-room/news-releases/apa-calls-for-end-to-armchair-psychiatry

Lee, B. X. (2017). *The dangerous case of Donald Trump: 27 psychiatrists and mental health experts assess a president.* New York, NY: St. Martin's Press.

Post, J. M. (1993). *The psychological assessment of political leaders, with profiles of Saddam Hussein and Bill Clinton.* Ann Arbor, MI: University of Michigan Press.

Post, J. M. (2015). *Narcissism and politics: Dreams of glory.* New York, NY: Cambridge University Press.

Post, J. M. (2015). *Dangerous charisma: The political psychology of Donald Trump and his followers.* New York, NY: Pegasus Books.

Stone, A. (2018, April 19). The psychiatrist's Goldwater rule in the Trump era. *Lawfare.* Retrieved from https://www.lawfaremedia.org/article/psychiatrists-goldwater-rule-trump-era

PARADOX AND POLITICAL ENDS OF THE GOLDWATER RULE

Surveying U.S. Mental Health Providers on their Role and Responsibility During Times of Perilous Politics

DENIS J. O'KEEFE, PH.D., L.C.S.W.

There is a kind of paradox in the American Psychiatric Association's March 2017 reauthorization and modification of the Goldwater Rule. While its purported aim is to avoid politicizing mental health, it inevitably reveals the inescapable link between mental health and politics. By restricting mental health professionals from sharing observations about public figures, the rule engages in a political act by limiting public access to expert knowledge. This 'silencing' benefits dangerous political movements, like right-wing nationalism, allowing it to flourish, and contributes to what American psychiatrist and author Robert J. Lifton (2017) calls "malignant normality" taking hold. It is this paradox that has led us to question potential underlying political motives of the APA's recent decision.

Our 2024 survey aims to provide insight into how mental health providers perceive these dynamics and unspoken political ends (O'Keefe et al, in press). This chapter will provide a brief overview of the purpose, findings, and implications of the survey designed to explore the opinions of a small but diverse group of U.S. mental health providers regarding their:

1. Knowledge of and expertise in addressing public health concerns in the political sphere.
2. Opinions on increasing educational requirements for engaging in political activities ethically.
3. Support for prioritizing societal health, such as a duty to warn, over the Goldwater Rule.
4. Experiences and repercussions of speaking out on political issues as a mental health provider.
5. The influence of authoritarian and political traits on support for the Goldwater Rule versus a duty to warn.

Context

There is a fundamental, yet thorny dialectic between the professional etiquette mental health experts owe to powerful public figures and their responsibility to society. This tension is articulated in the code of ethics of all mental health professions, the Declaration of Geneva, and the Hippocratic Oath, often framed as a "duty to warn" regarding threats to societal health. The Declaration of Geneva, adopted by the World Medical Association in 1948, represents a modern iteration of the Hippocratic Oath. Its inception followed a critical examination of Nazi Germany's medicalization of political violence (Lifton, 1986). The Nuremberg trials demonstrated that silently "following orders" is not a viable defense for unethical actions. The use of medical violence is a clear example of an authoritarian process (Adorno, et al., 1982; Lifton, 1986), whereby professionals abdicate their judgment and decision-making, effectively displacing moral or ethical reasoning or critique. This process, thoroughly analyzed in Robert J. Lifton's book *The Nazi Doctors* (1986) and revisited in his foreword to *The Dangerous Case of Donald Trump* (2017), underscores the perils of medical professionals relinquishing moral judgment. Lifton's work highlights the dangers of how such abdication can lead to the normalization of political violence, urging mental health experts to be 'witnessing professionals,' actively calling out potential societal harm.

The health and integrity of democratic societies depends on an informed public and a free, independent press playing crucial roles in discerning truth from the discourses of power and educating a voting public. Authoritarian regimes with charismatic leaders rise by controlling information, exalting nationalism, ethnocentrism, and militarism while "othering" marginalized groups. The label of "enemies of the state" justifies the silencing and persecution of critical voices. This tactic has been repeatedly used throughout history. Today, the global resurgence of right-wing nationalist movements has raised alarm among mental health experts, who are increasingly concerned about the psychological and societal impacts of authoritarianism (Osborne et al., 2023; Lee, 2020). Donald Trump and the MAGA movement may exemplify this trend, but a few examples beyond American leaders include Vladimir Putin of Russia, Kim Jong-un of North Korea, Xi Jinping of China, Recep Tayyip Erdoğan of Turkey, Benjamin Netanyahu of Israel, Javier Milei in Argentina, and Jair Bolsonaro in Brazil, to name just a few. In European democracies, Marine Le Pen and more recently Jordan Bardella in France, Giorgia Meloni in Italy, the Sweden Democrats with its neo-Nazi origins, the Geert Wilders in the Netherlands, Alternative for Germany Party and its leader Alice Weidel in Germany, and Viktor Orban of Hungary, among others.

The silencing of mental health professions serves the information control needs of populist autocrats. The American Psychiatric Association's stance on avoiding the politicization of mental health, paradoxically, was established within an increasingly politicized system shaped by right-wing nationalism, making mental health professionals unwitting collaborators. Silence, in this context, has an unstated function serving a political end. Our hypothesis explores the link between political orientation and attitudes toward a duty to warn, suggesting that authoritarian traits, often associated with right-wing ideology, mediate this relationship, enabling the expression of authoritarian impulses under the guise of political acts like forced silence. (O'Keefe et al., in press).

Survey Findings

In the context of increasing concern over political risks to democracy, and aligned with the mission of the World Mental Health Coalition led by Bandy Lee, our 2024 survey was conducted to explore the perceived role of mental health experts in assessing the risks that political movements and leaders can pose to democracy and societal stability. 118 professionals representing the subspecialties of psychology, social work, psychiatry, mental health counseling and marriage and family therapy responded to the survey. From the outset, we sought to understand whether these experts have the desire and believed they possess knowledge and expertise to speak out about public health concerns in the political sphere. The responses suggest that they do and with high confidence. Roughly 96% of respondents felt knowledgeable enough to speak out on public health concerns in the political sphere, with over 80% feeling moderately to extremely knowledgeable. Further, around 90% believed political psychological models should be included in clinical training programs, with roughly 74% indicating strong support.

When questioned whether they have personally spoken out on societal issues from a psychological vantage point, over 90% say they have, with over 70% doing so in the range of "moderately regularly" to "always". Despite this confidence, when those who do speak out were asked if they experienced any forms of retaliation, all respondents indicated some level of retaliation, with 27% reporting "sometimes" and 43% indicating high levels of "often" and "always". These striking numbers support the assertion that normative, 'silencing' pressures are present, begging future research to explore the forms and quality of retaliation experienced, the extent to which it impacts the content, and when and where opinions are shared.

It is no surprise, given the percentage of those speaking out, that only 8% of participants showed relative support for the Goldwater rule over a duty to warn. The highest scores were for survey items measuring support for holding professional associations responsible for disinformation; concern regarding political leaders' rhetoric as it impacts public health; mental health professionals' responsibility to public health in the political domain; and support for a public forum for mental health experts to address political behavior that has negative public health consequences. The findings also indicated that at least for these participants, increasing conservative political orientation and authoritarian traits predicted Goldwater favoritism over a duty to warn. Following that 'silence' has overwhelmingly supported the political ends of the Republican party, which has been increasingly influenced by a right-wing nationalist agenda, political orientation significantly mediated authoritarianism, supporting the claim that political beliefs are utilized as justification for the expression of authoritarian behavior such as 'silencing.'

Conclusion

When given the means and opportunity, mental health experts are able and willing to disrupt ideologically-driven justifications of dangerous political movements. This is especially crucial in confronting 'malignant normalizing' discourses that seek to legitimize autocratic leaders. However, the American Psychiatric Association (APA) has implemented measures that effectively ubiquitously silence 'witnessing professionals.'

The APA's motives are questionable, given a refusal to entertain a debate on the subject despite the unpopularity of the 2017 Goldwater rule amendments among mental health experts across the professions. The punitive implementation of these amendments has further raised concerns (O'Keefe et al., in press). While the APA claims to depoliticize mental health, their actions have revealed a fundamental paradox: By denying the political context of their decision, they have inadvertently produced profoundly political consequences.

This silencing of mental health professionals inadvertently serves right-wing nationalist agendas that seek to control information. As a result, these professionals have become unwitting participants violating the Geneva Pledge and their commitment to societal health. Meanwhile, media outlets have grown increasingly concerned about potential litigation.

It is heartening to note that most surveyed professionals in this study consider the duty to warn a higher ethical responsibility than adherence to the Goldwater rule. However, it is not coincidental that those supporting the rule tend to have more conservative political leanings and display authoritarian personality traits. This correlation should prompt us to question the unspoken agenda behind the APA's Goldwater Amendment.

Denis J. O'Keefe, PhD, LCSW, is a Professor of Social Work at New York University, where he teaches graduate and doctoral courses on social policy and the intersection of social theory and clinical practice. His research focuses on the psychology of ideology and development of a psychological social policy analytic model. He is a Research Associate of the Psychohistory Forum and the Clinic Director of the Family Resource Center in Highland Falls, NY, where he maintains his private practice. He is a past President of the International Psychohistorical Association and current Director of Research of the World Mental Health Coalition.

References

Lee, B. X. (2017). *The Dangerous Case of Donald Trump: 27 Psychiatrists and mental health experts assess a president.* New York, NY: Saint Martin's Press.

Lee, B. X. (2020). *Profile of a Nation: Trump's Mind, America's Soul.* New York, NY: World Mental Health Coalition.

Lifton, R. J. (1986). *The Nazi Doctors: Medical Killing and the Psychology of Genocide.* New York, NY: Basic Books.

Lifton, R. J. (2017). Our witness to malignant normality. In B. X. Lee, ed., *The dangerous case of Donald Trump: 27 psychiatrists and mental health experts assess a president.* New York, NY: Saint Martin's Press.

O'Keefe, D., Lee, B. X., McGinnis, K., McCullough, A. & Krenn, C. (in press). Silence vs. bearing witness: Mental health professionals' responsibility to society in a time of perilous politics. *Journal for the Advancement of Scientific Psychoanalytic Empirical Research.*

Osborne, D., Costello, T. H., Duckitt, J., & Sibly, C. (2023). The psychological causes and societal consequences of authoritarianism." *Nature Reviews Psychology* 2, 220-232. World Medical Association (1948). Declaration of Geneva. Geneva, Switzerland: World Medical Association https://www.wma.net/policies-post/wma-declaration-of-Geneva/.

PART 4
AESCULAPIUS
(GOD OF HEALING)

UNBRIDLED AND EXTREME PRESENT HEDONISM

How the [Former] Leader of the Free World has Proven Time and Again He is Unfit for Duty

Philip Zimbardo, Ph.D., and Rosemary Sword

(This is an excerpt of their original essay submitted in 2017, still relevant today, reprinted here with permission.)

The following is provided as background to assist in understanding how we have come to the conclusion that Donald Trump displays the most threatening time perspective profile— that of an extreme present hedonist—and is therefore "unfit for duty."

Time Perspective Theory and Therapy (TPT)

We are all familiar with the three main time zones: the past, the present, and the future. In a TPT, these time zones are divided into subsets: *past positive* and *past negative*; *present hedonism* and *present fatalism*; and *future positive* and *future negative*. When one of these time perspectives is too heavily weighed, we can lose out on what's really happening now and/or lose sight of what could be happening in our future, causing us to be unsteady, unbalanced, or temporally biased.

Being out of balance in this way also shades the way we think, as well as negatively impacts our daily decision-making process. For instance, if you are stuck in a past negative experience, you might think that from now on everything that happens to you will be negative, so why even bother planning for your future, because it's just going to continue to be the same old bad stuff. Or if you are an extreme present hedonist adrenaline junky intent on spiking your adrenal glands, then you might engage in risky behaviors that unintentionally endanger yourself or others because you are living in the moment and not thinking about the future consequences of today's actions. If you are out of balance in your future time perspective, constantly thinking and worrying about all the things you have to do, or must do on your endless to-do list, you might forget or miss out on the everyday, wonderful things happening in your life and the lives of your loved ones in the here and now.

6 Main Time Perspectives in TPT

1. *Past positive* people focus on the good things that have happened.
2. *Past negative* people focus on all the things that went wrong in the past.
3. *Present hedonistic* people live in the moment, seeking pleasure, novelty, sensation, and avoiding pain.
4. *Present fatalistic* people feel that planning for future decisions is not necessary because predetermined fate plays the guiding role in one's life.
5. *Future positive* people plan for the future and trust that their decision will work out.
6. *Future negative* people feel the future is fatalistic, apocalyptic, or have no future-orientation.

Present Hedonism and Arrested Emotional Development

As mentioned above, *present hedonists* live and act in the moment, frequently with little to no thought of the future, or the consequences of their actions. Most children and teenagers are present hedonists; each day they build on past experiences, but their concept of the future is still under development. People suffering from arrested emotional development, usually caused by a childhood trauma, are also present hedonists. The ability to emotionally mature beyond the age of trauma without therapy is difficult to impossible. When they reach adulthood, they may be able to hide their lack of emotional maturity for periods of time, and then when in a stressful situation, they revert to behaving the emotional age they were when they were first traumatized. Depending on the degree that the childhood trauma has affected the person suffering from arrested emotional development, they may find that over time, their present hedonistic time perspective has morphed into extreme present hedonism.

Without proper individual assessment, we are only best-guessing as to whether or not Donald Trump may suffer from arrested emotional development, which may or may not be a factor in the cause of his extreme present hedonism. But due to the extensive amount of print and video media exposing his bully-type behavior, his immature remarks about sex, and his childlike need for constant attention, we can speculate that the traumatizing event was when he was sent away to military school at the age of thirteen. According to one of his biographers, Michael D'Antonio, "He (Trump) was essentially banished from the family home. He hadn't known anything but living with his family in a luxurious setting, and all of a sudden, he's sent away."[1] This would help explain his pubescent default setting when confronted by others.

Extreme Present Hedonism

An *extreme present hedonist* will say or do anything at any time for purposes of self-aggrandizement and to shield themselves from previous— usually negatively perceived— activities with *no* thought of the future or the effect of their actions. And with a measure of paranoia, which is the norm, extreme present hedonism is the most unpredictable and perilous time perspective due to its "action" component. Here's how it works:

The *extreme present hedonist*'s impulsive thought leads to an impulsive action that can cause them to dig in their heels when confronted with the consequences of that action. If the person is in a position of power, then others scramble to either deny or find ways to back up the original impulsive action. In normal, day-to-day life, this impulsiveness leads to misunderstandings, lying, and toxic relationships. In the case of Donald Trump, an impulsive thought may unleash a stream of tweets or verbal remarks (the action), which spurs others to try to fulfill—or deny—Trump's thoughtless action.

Donald Trump's Extreme Present Hedonistic Quotes

It could be argued that almost anyone can be presented in a negative light when scrutinized and quoted out of context. However, when one runs for the highest office in the land, and then wins the prize, such scrutiny is expected. In the case of Donald Trump, there is a rich trove of recorded examples that give us a strong picture of the inner workings of his unbalanced psyche. The following well-known quotes compiled by Michael Kruse and Noah Weiland for *Politico Magazine* ("Donald Trump's Greatest Self Contradictions," May 5, 2016)— some of them overlap into multiple categories—

illustrate his extreme present hedonistic penchant for off-roading from his script and/or saying or tweeting whatever pops into his mind, making things up, repeating fake news, or simply lying:

Dehumanization:
- "Sometimes, part of making a deal is denigrating your competition." *The Art of the Deal*, 1987.
- "When Mexico sends its people, they're not sending their best…They're sending people that have a lot of problems, and they're bringing those problems with us. They're bringing drugs. They're bringing crime. They're rapists. And some, I assume, are good people." Republican Presidential Acceptance speech, June 16, 2015.
- "Written by a nice reporter. Now the poor guy. You ought to see this guy." Rally in South Carolina; as Trump said these things about journalist Serge Kovaleski, he contorted his face and moved his arms and hands around awkwardly. Kovaleski has arthrogryposis, a congenital condition that can limit joint movement or lock limbs in place. November 24, 2015.

Lying:
- "'Made in America? @BarackObama called his 'birthplace' Hawaii 'here in Asia.'" Tweet, November 18, 2011.
- "I watched when the World Trade Center came tumbling down…And I watched in Jersey City, New Jersey, where thousands and thousands of people were cheering as that building was coming down. Thousands of people were cheering." At a rally in Birmingham, Alabama, November 21, 2015.
The next day, "This Week" host George Stephanopoulos pointed out that "the police say that didn't happen." Trump insisted otherwise: "It was on television. I saw it happen."
- "In addition to winning the Electoral College in a landslide, I won the popular vote if you deduct the millions of people who voted illegally." Tweet, November 27, 2016.

Misogyny:
- "You could see there was blood coming out of her eyes. Blood coming out of

her—wherever." During a CNN interview, in regards to Megyn Kelly, following the previous night's Fox News debate co-moderated by Kelly, in which Kelly asked Trump about his misogynistic treatment of women, August 7, 2015.

- "Look at that face! Would anybody vote for that? Can you imagine that the face of our next president? ... I mean, she's a woman, and I'm not supposed to say bad things, but really, folks, come on. Are we serious?" In a *Rolling Stone* interview in regards to Republican presidential candidate Carly Fiorina, September 9, 2015.

- "When you're a star, they let you do it. You can do anything ...Grab them by the p***y ... You can do anything." Off-camera remarks recorded in 2005 by Access Hollywood and published by the Washington Post in October 2016.

Paranoia:

- "The world is a vicious and brutal place. We think we're civilized. In truth, it's a cruel world and people are ruthless. They act nice to your face, but underneath they're out to kill you...Even your friends are out to get you: they want your job, they want your house, they want your money, they want your wife, and they even want your dog. Those are your friends; your enemies are even worse!" *Trump: Think Big,* 2007.

- "My motto is 'Hire the best people, and don't trust them.'" *Trump: Think Big,* 2007.

- "If you have smart people working for you, they'll try to screw you if they think they can do better without you." *Daily Mail,* October 30, 2010.

Racism:

- "You haven't been called, go back to Univision." Dismissing Latino reporter Jorge Ramos at an Iowa rally, August 2015.

- "Donald J. Trump is calling for a total and complete shutdown of Muslims entering the United States." At a rally in Charleston, S.C., December 2015.

- "Look at my African American over here. Look at him." At a campaign appearance in California, June 2016.

Self-aggrandizement:

- "I'm, like, a really smart person." During an interview in Phoenix, Arizona,

July 11, 2015.

   ● "It's very hard for them to attack me on my looks, because I'm so good look-ing." During an interview, August 7, 2015.

   ● "I'm speaking with myself, No. 1, because I have a very good brain and I've said a lot of things. … My primary consultant is myself." MSNBC interview, March 16, 2016.

In Donald Trump, we have a frightening Venn diagram consisting of three circles; the first is extreme present hedonism, the second narcissism, and the third bully behavior. These three circles converge and meet in the middle to create the perfect storm of an impulsive, immature, incompetent person who, when in the position of ultimate power, easily slides into the role of tyrant, complete with family members sitting at his prover-bial "ruling table." Like a fledgling dictator, he plants psychological seeds of treachery that reinforce already negative attitudes in sections of our population.

The Results

In line with the principles of Regents of the University of California, 17 Cal. 3d 425 (1976)— known as the "Tarasoff doctrine"— it was, and continues to be the responsibility of mental health professionals to warn the citizens of the United States as well as the world of the potentially devastating effects of such an extreme present hedo-nistic world leader, one with enormous power at his disposal. As a whole, mental health professionals have failed in the duty to warn, in a timely manner, not only the public but also government officials, about the dangers of President Donald Trump. Pre-election articles and interviews intent on cautioning the masses fell on deaf ears, perhaps in part because the media did not afford the concerned mental health professionals appropriate coverage, perhaps because some citizens discount the value of mental health and have thrown a thick blanket of stigma on the profession, or perhaps because we did not stand united. Whatever the reason, it's not too late to follow through.

   Our nation as a whole can be viewed like a person in that when psychologically unbalanced, *everything* teeters and can fall apart if we don't realize a change must occur. We wonder how far-reaching— in terms of our society as well as in time— the actions of our unbalanced president have affected and will continue to affect us as individuals, communities, a nation, and a planet. We believe that Donald Trump is the most danger-ous man in the world; a powerful leader of a powerful nation who can order missile firing at another nation because of his (or his family member's) personal distress at seeing sad scenes of people having been gassed to death. We shudder to imagine repeated escalations of such personal emotions into broader lethal confrontations with HIS enemies.

We are gravely concerned about his abrupt, capricious one hundred- and eighty-degree shifts and how these displays of instability have the potential to be unconscionably dangerous to the point of causing catastrophe, and not only for the citizens of the U.S. Two examples that are particularly troubling are: 1) repeatedly lavishing praise of FBI director James Comey's handling of Hillary Clinton's emails during the campaign and then suddenly, and abusively, firing Comey, supposedly for the same reason that had garnered such praise (but apparently because of Comey's investigation into the Russia investigation); 2) constant pre- and post-campaign rhetoric that NATO was obsolete and then unexpectedly stating NATO is necessary and acceptable. As is Trump's extreme present hedonistic way, he's "chumming" for war, possibly for the most selfish of reasons—to change the subject from the Russia investigations. And if another unbalanced world leader takes the bait, he will need the formerly "obsolete" and now essential NATO to back him up.

But we as individuals don't have to follow the leader down a path that leads us in the wrong direction—off a cliff and into the pit of past mistakes. We can stand where we are at this moment in history and face forward into a brighter future *we* create. We can start by looking for the good in each other and the common ground we share.

In the midst of the terrorist attacks on places of worship and cemeteries mentioned earlier, something wonderful emerged from the ashes: the spirit of overwhelming goodness in humanity. Jews and Muslims united to collaborate in the wake of attacks. They held fundraisers to help each other repair and rebuild; they shared places of worship to hold gatherings and services; and offered loving support while facing hatred. Through these acts of compassion and observing ordinary people engaging in acts of every day heroism, we are witnessing the best aspects of humanity. *That's* us! *That's* the United States of America!

A final suggestion for our governmental leaders: Corporations and companies vet their prospective employees. This vetting process frequently includes psychological testing in the form of exams or quizzes to help the employer make more informed hiring decisions and determine if the prospective employee is honest and/or would be a good fit for the company. These tests are used on employees ranging from department store sales to high-level executive positions. Isn't it time the same is required for the candidates of the most important job in the world?

Philip Zimbardo, Ph.D., Professor Emeritus at Stanford University, is a scholar, educator and researcher. Dr. Zimbardo is perhaps best known for his landmark Stanford prison study. Among his more than 500 publications are the bestseller The Lucifer Effect, *and such notable psychology textbooks as* Psychology: Core Concepts, 8th edition *and* Psychology and Life, *now in its 20th edition. He is founder and president of The Heroic Imagination Project (heroicimagination.org), a worldwide nonprofit teaching people of all ages how to take wise and effective action in challenging situations. He also continues to research the effects of time perspectives and time perspective therapy.*

Rosemary Sword is codeveloper of Time Perspective Therapy and coauthor of The Time Cure *(in English, German, Polish, Chinese, and Russian),* The Time Cure Therapist Guidebook, *Wiley, 2013;* Time Perspective Therapy: Transforming Zimbardo's Temporal Theory into Clinical Practice, Time Perspective Theory, *Springer, 2015;* Living and Loving Better, *McFarland, November 2017; and* Time Perspective Therapy: An Evolutionary Therapy for PTSD, *McFarland, to be announced. Sword and Zimbardo write a popular column for* PsychologyToday.com *and contribute to both* AppealPower.com, *a European Union online journal, and* Psychology in Practice, *a new Polish psychological journal. She is also developer of Aetas: Mind Balancing Apps discoveraetas.com).*

References

Schwartzman, P. & Miller, M. E., (2016, June 22). Confident. incorrigible. bully: Little Donny was a lot like candidate Donald Trump. *The Washington Post*. Retrieved from https://www.washingtonpost.com/lifestyle/style/young-donald-trump-military-school/2016/06/22/f0b3b164-317c-11e6-8758-d58e76e11b12_story.html?utm_term=.961fefcee834

Zimbardo, P. & Boyd, J. (2009). *The Time Paradox*. New York: Atria.

Zimbardo, P., Sword, Ri. & Sword, Ro. (2012). *The Time Cure*. San Francisco, CA: Wiley.

Kruse, M. & Weiland, N. (2016, May 5). Donald Trump's greatest self-contradictions. *Politico Magazine*. Retrieved from http://www.politico.com/magazine/story/2016/05/donald-trump-2016-contradictions-213869

THE DANGEROUS CASE OF THE AMERICAN PEOPLE

Prudence Gourguechon, M.D.

Would you hire Donald Trump to be a teacher in your preschool? How about treasurer on your synagogue board? I don't think so. The reason you would not is that he has shown himself to be unfit to carry responsibility for institutions or peoples' lives. My colleagues and I made a sound case for that in *The Dangerous Case of Donald Trump*. Events that have happened since only confirm our observations and predictions.

But what haunts me now is something different. It is the dangerous case of the American people. How can we explain the current poll numbers—that Trump has a 44.5% approval rating as of this writing? How do we explain the fact that nearly 44% of the American voting public plans to vote for this unfit person, this convicted felon, this disorganized, selfish, untrustworthy, uncaring conman?

I want to tease apart some of the psychological reasons behind what otherwise seems inexplicable. There are, of course, profound political, economic and sociological reasons, as well as a deeply consequential shift in our means of getting information from algorithm-dictated silos. These contributors are powerful and deserve exploration by experts in those fields. But each of the broad political and economic forces achieves its impact in part by creating intense emotional states that influence voters' decision-making.

The powerful psychological forces at work include fear, resistance to change, regression, humiliation and helplessness, groupthink, the defense mechanisms of disavowal and identification with the aggressor, and the activation of primitive transferences.

One crucial caveat—all of the regressive, destructive psychological forces explained briefly below are part of every person's psychological repertoire. The are not limited to any one demographic. This is where people go when feeling threatened.

206

Fear and Resistance to Change

These two factors work hand in hand, amplifying each other in a negative feedback loop. The more you resist change, the more frightened you become. The more frightened you become, the more you fight change. Our current moment in history is experienced by most as a time of massively heightened change. Changing social mores and behavior, climate change, migration, radically new ways of being in community and communicating and decreasing identification with traditional social structures combine to create a deep sense of threat for many people. This makes people vulnerable to psychological manipulation.

Regression

This perpetually stressful and unsettled state of mind leads to *psychological regression*—a slide towards a more primitive kind of mental functioning, where critical thinking is overridden by emotion, judgment is faulty, emotion overrides thinking, and the dangerous defense mechanisms of disavowal, identification with the aggressor, and primitive transferences are mobilized. Greed, a human potential that is always present, is likely to surge during regressed states.

Humiliation and Helplessness

The overload of change described above creates an internal atmosphere of helplessness.

Current historical circumstances tilt towards creating a sense of humiliation and helplessness in some groups. Paradigmatic is the white working-class Trump voter whose grandfather had a good job in a steel mill, but who sees a truncated economic future for himself. Humiliation and helplessness are powerful negative emotions that can lead to desperate attempts to feel better at any cost, including scapegoating, identifying with a bully, and joining efforts to isolate and divide.

Groupthink

Groupthink is a psychological trap to which we are all vulnerable. When we are part of a group where strongly held views predominate, it becomes increasingly difficult to maintain an independent point of view. Social pressure and internal pressure to conform are extremely powerful. Bucking the group's point of view leads to painful isolation and self-doubt. This is not as simple a matter of hiding one's differences. Groupthink actually changes minds, erasing minority opinions in favor of conformity.

Disavowal

Part of human psychology is the employment of defense mechanisms to help cope with unwelcome or negative emotions or thoughts. For the most part these defense mechanisms play a positive role and adaptive role, allowing us to set aside fears that otherwise might immobilize us. Disavowal is the defense that allows you to get in a car and drive despite the knowledge that you actually could get in a fatal accident. You mentally set aside or disavow the risks of automobile travel in order to get on with your life. Disavowal permits you to drain unwelcome truths of influence and effect. A woman can vote for Trump because disavowal allows the facts of his multiple sexual assaults, unfaithfulness, and bullying and insulting women to be mentally pushed away behind a wall. A veteran can vote for Trump because the fact of his mocking of John McCain and diminishing the Medal of Honor can be exiled by disavowal to a corner of his mind.

Identification with the Aggressor

Identification with the aggressor is another defense mechanism that is employed, especially when people are dealing with feelings of helplessness. In this situation, instead of feeling oppressed or uncared for by the actions of an aggressive leader or bully, individuals identify with him, telling themselves that they can take part in his perceived strength and mastery.

Primitive transferences

Transference is another ubiquitous part of mental life. We all tend to experience authority figures in our life through a lens shaped by early experiences with our parents and others who cared for us. Teachers, clergy, doctors, and political leaders all become stand-ins for parental figures, and we judge them by their ability to stand in for a "good mother" or "good father." States of regression lead to more psychologically primitive transferences. In the dangerous case of the American people, Trump elicits a powerful strongman transference. He positions himself as the ultimate powerful father who is omnipotent, omniscient and, in a strange way, loving. He said in his first campaign, "Only I can fix it," a brief phrase that efficiently accomplished two aims: intensifying fears that something essential is threatened, or broken, and asserting his role as an omnipotent strong man who will bring redemption and repair. That both of these contentions are absurd is irrelevant. He successfully captures and plays on fleeting emotional truth and makes it determinative.

What can heal the American people?

Given these psychological forces, how can we shift the American narrative?

The relationship between the leader and the led is complex. Human beings are in part, though not entirely, herd animals. Famously, 1500 sheep did follow a lone leader who jumped off a cliff in a town in Turkey in 2005; 450 perished, and the livelihood of a small town with them. Removal of a pathological leader from the scene, one who stokes fear, encourages regressive hyper-emotional responses, undermines critical thinking and decimates public trust, would allow space for regaining emotional equilibrium and psychologically constructive processes. One of the great psychological tragedies of our recent political history, to my mind, is the collusion of Republican leaders in Trump's mismanagement of the American mind. If the likes of Lindsey Graham, Nicky Haley, Marco Rubio and others had stuck with their original public dismay about Donald Trump's ineptness and psychological dangerousness despite personal cost, the capacity of the American public to recover from their political psychological illness would have been greatly enhanced.

To affect a reversal of these destructive and regressive psychological trends, a key tactic is to accept the emotions as real and powerful. If you know what to do about them, say so clearly and directly. If you don't know, acknowledge that and say you'll work through it together. One of the pillars of Trump's psychological success is that he acknowledged the pervasive sense of threat and alienation much of the populace feels.

Combating helplessness and hopelessness is essential. Vice President Harris and Governor Walz, with the unexpected joy and optimism evident early in their campaign, quickly made inroads against hopelessness. When people feel hopeful and less helpless, they are less likely to function at a regressed, hyper-emotional level.

Tim Walz's persona as The Coach, strong, nurturing and fair, offers an alternative paternal transference figure to Trump's strongman who leads by humiliation.

Humor might be the best weapon to confront fear of change. Trump's language blatantly stokes fear of change. "Millions of people are crossing the border to take Black jobs," he asserted, also claiming repeatedly that cities are disasters and hellholes and institutions are corrupt. Saying this is a set of lies is frustratingly ineffective. But who can forget Simone Biles saying at the Paris Olympics, "I love my Black job."

Manifesting optimism, hope and humor implicitly acknowledges the psychological forces in play, but transforms them from destructive and regressive ones to growth-promoting and community-fostering influences.

Prudence Gourguechon, M.D., is a past President of the American Psychoanalytic Association (APsaA). Following a 40-year career as a psychiatrist and psychoanalyst, she currently works as a consultant on the psychology of business, advising executives on leader assessment and the psychological underpinnings of business relationships and decisions. She also serves as a psychiatric expert witness and litigation consultant. She founded APsaA's Service Members and Veterans Initiative and spearheaded a successful effort to include military history in the AMA's Current Procedural Terminology (CPT) Code's guide to social history. A Forbes.com senior contributor on leadership strategy, she can be contacted through her website, www.prudencegourguechonmd.com.

References

The Hill. August 24, 2024

Fivethirtyeight.com August 24, 2024

A CLINICAL CASE FOR THE DANGEROUSNESS OF DONALD J. TRUMP REVISITED

Diane Jhueck, L.M.H.C.

It has been seven years since a group of professionals in the field of mental health came together with a sense of urgency about the dangerousness of Donald Trump as President of the United States. Together, we wrote *The Dangerous Case of Donald Trump*, hoping to warn our country about the grave issues we were seeing, through the lens of our particular areas of expertise.

My involvement with this book began with an online petition that I wrote, which was ultimately signed by about 80 licensed mental health professionals, asking that Trump be given a mental health assessment for dangerousness in New York State. This was where he was still residing, as he had initially refused to move into the White House. While creating this petition, I reviewed public records of recordings of Trump as well as interviews from witnesses to his behaviors. Such evidence is often used in the investigation phase of a petition for civil commitment. It can be argued that there is more existing data to determine diagnosis on Trump than most mental health specialists have available to them for their own patients.

The specific disorders indicated by this review in 2017 were as follows:

a. Antisocial Personality Disorder (pervasive pattern of violation of the rights of others, deceitful, impulsive, irritable/aggressive, consistent failure to honor financial obligations);

b. Narcissistic Personality Disorder (pervasive grandiosity, need for admiration, lack of empathy, expectation of being viewed as superior without commensurate achievements, unreasonable sense of entitlement, interpersonally exploitative, arrogant, envy driven);

       c. Histrionic Personality Disorder (pervasive excessive emotionality and attention seeking, distress if not center of attention, interactions often characterized by inappropriate sexual behavior, labile, speech is impressionistic and lacks detail, self-dramatizing/theatrical, easily influenced by others, considers relationships to be more intimate than they are).

       d. A high likelihood of a major neurological diagnosis was indicated by Trump's chronological age, his biological father's diagnosis of Alzheimer's Disease, apparent covering by his three oldest children, who have assumed historically unprecedented roles related to his Presidency, amnestic presentation, and behavioral variants as well as language variants would indicate the need to rule out Alzheimer's Disease.

It is now 2024, and Trump provides most of us with a near-daily display of all the symptoms described above. This includes a notable decrease in his cognitive function.

It has become common to describe Trump as having "Malignant Narcissism." However, this is not a formal diagnosis in our profession and, in my view, distracts from one of his significant dangers to us—his likely Antisocial Personality Disorder. Ishita Aggarwal writes, "Antisocial personality disorder (ASPD)…is a mental illness that is characterized by a reckless disregard for social norms, impulsive behaviour, an inability to experience guilt, and a low tolerance for frustration. Individuals with ASPD exhibit an inflated sense of self-worth and possess a superficial charm, traits that often aid their attempts to exploit and violate the rights of others." She continues, "Criminal behaviour is frequently associated with ASPD," (Aggarwal 2013). While roughly 5% or less of the general population has ASPD, it is the most common mental health disorder among people who are incarcerated. A Cambridge University review of recent studies on the subject determined that "… the prevalence of ASPD ranges between 0.6% and 4.3% in men (which is significantly higher than in women)….The prevalence of ASPD among prisoners is 55% among men and 31% among women," (Howard and Duggan 2022). It is highly likely that Trump has a mental illness that removes his personal choice concerning whether to engage in criminal acts and harm others. With this diagnosis, Trump is effectively a criminal by nature.

Of note, the only professional to examine and evaluate Hitler (to whom Trump is often compared) determined in 1923 that Hitler was, "...a hysteric and pathological psychopath," (Kaplan 2020). These diagnoses equate to Histrionic Personality Disorder and Antisocial Personality Disorder.

Ignoring other disturbing news (such as the Project 2025 document), and highlighting just one example of many indicating that Trump is even more dangerous than he was when elected to office previously, consider the Supreme Court immunity determination. The Justices write:

The indictment next alleges that Trump and his co-conspirators "attempted to enlist the Vice President to use his ceremonial role at the January 6 certification proceeding to fraudulently alter the election results" (App. 187, Indictment 10(d)). In particular, the indictment alleges several conversations in which Trump pressured the Vice President to reject States' legitimate electoral votes or send them back to state legislatures for review. Whenever the President and Vice President discuss their official responsibilities, they engage in official conduct...The indictment's allegations that Trump attempted to pressure the Vice President to take particular acts in connection with his role at the certification proceeding thus involve official conduct, and Trump is at least presumptively immune from prosecution for such conduct. (Supreme Court of the United States 2024, Syllabus, Pp. 17-19, ii).

Even without this decision, his access to the nuclear codes already made him an existential threat to all humankind. This new determination would truly render him the most dangerous person on the planet, should he again assume the presidency.

The mass delusion that has been displayed by Trump followers, sycophants, and those using his very apparent array of mental illnesses for their own gain, has been extremely troubling in regard to its hold on our socio-political system for close to a decade. The magnitude of the surge of hope that is currently spreading through that same system, consequent to Biden's highly unusual personal sacrifice and the refreshingly mentally healthy Harris/Walz ticket, will be interesting to follow over the course of the next few months and into the future. There may well be new data to mine on the topic of what is required for large and complex political systems to heal.

Diane Jhueck, L.M.H.C., has operated a private therapy practice for almost 30 years. She recently retired from performing evaluations for in-

voluntary commitment on individuals presenting as a danger to self or others due to mental illness. In a previous social justice career, she was a women's program specialist at the United Nations in New York City. She founded The Women's and Children's Free Restaurant, an empowerment project that has now been in operation just under 40 years. She directed agencies and programs addressing food aid, domestic violence, apartheid, low-income housing, and LGBTQ rights.

References

Aggarwal, I. (2013). Vol 5 No. 09, pp. 1-2. The Role of Antisocial Personality Disorder and Antisocial Behavior in Crime. *Inquiries Journal Social Sciences, Arts, & Humanities.*

American Psychiatric Association. (2022). *Diagnostic and Statistical Manual of Mental Disorders. 5th ed.*

Howard, R. & Duggan, C. (2022, January 20). *The Epidemiology of Antisocial Personality Disorder.* Chapter 5. Published online by Cambridge University Press.

Kaplan, R. M. (2020, June 25). Alois Maria Ott: I was Hitler's Psychologist. *Psychiatric Times.*

Supreme Court of the United States. (2024, July 1). Trump v. United States. Certiorari to the United States Court of Appeals for the District of Columbia Circuit, No. 23-939. Argued April 25, 2024-Decided July 1, 2024.

PROTECTING THE NUCLEAR FOOTBALL
The Twenty–fifth Amendment and Legislative Solutions

NANETTE GARTRELL, M.D. AND DEE MOSBACHER, M.D., PH.D.

(Portions of this chapter were originally published in The Dangerous Case of Donald Trump: 37 Psychiatrists and Mental Health Experts Assess a President.*)*

In 1994, President Jimmy Carter lamented our inability to ensure that the person entrusted with the nuclear arsenal is mentally and physically capable of fulfilling that responsibility (Carter, 1994). Throughout U.S. history, presidents have suffered from serious psychiatric or medical conditions, most of which were unknown to the public. A review of U.S. presidential office holders from 1776-1974 revealed that 49% of the 37 presidents met criteria that suggested psychiatric disorders (Davidson, Connor, and Swartz, 2006). For example, Presidents Pierce and Lincoln had symptoms of depression (Davidson, Connor, and Swartz 2006), Nixon and Johnson, paranoia (Glaister, 2008; Goodwin, 1988), and Reagan, dementia (Berisha et al., 2015). President Wilson experienced a massive stroke that resulted in severely impaired cognitive functioning (Weinstein, 1981). Mr. Trump's hostile, impulsive, provocative, suspicious, and erratic conduct has posed a grave threat to our national security (Barbaro, 2016; DelReal and Gearan, 2016; Kendall, 2016; Miller and Jaffe, 2017; Montanaro, 2024; Pelosi, 2024; Reilly, 2016; Sebastian, 2016; TIME Staff, 2024; Wagner, 2017; Zaur, 2017). Although military personnel who are responsible for relaying nuclear orders must undergo rigorous mental health and medical evaluations that assess psychological, financial, and medical fitness for duty (Colón-Francia and Fortner, 2014; Osnos, 2017), there is no such requirement for their commander-in-chief.

The Twenty-fifth Amendment to the U.S. Constitution addresses presidential disability and succession (Cornell University Law School, 2017). Section 4 of this amendment has never been invoked to evaluate whether a standing president is fit to serve. We call on Congress to pass legislation to ensure that presidential and vice-presidential candidates are evaluated by a professional panel before the general election, and that the sitting president and vice-president are assessed on an annual basis. We also recommend that panel members receive all medical and mental health reports on the president and vice-president, with the authorization to request any additional evaluations the panel deems necessary.

Our specific recommendations are as follows:

1. Under Section 4 of the Twenty-fifth Amendment to the U.S. Constitution, Congress should constitute an independent, nonpartisan panel of mental health and medical experts to evaluate every president's capability to fulfill the responsibilities of the office.

2. The panel should consist of three neuropsychiatrists (one clinical, one academic, and one military), one clinical psychologist, one neurologist, and two internists.

3. Panel members should be nominated by the nonpartisan, nongovernmental National Academy of Medicine (Abrams, 1999).

4. The experts should serve six-year terms, with a provision that one member per year will rotate off and be replaced (Abrams, 1999).

5. Congress should enact legislation to authorize this panel to perform comprehensive mental health and medical evaluations of the president and vice-president on an annual basis. This legislation should require the panel to evaluate all presidential and vice-presidential candidates. The panel should also be empowered to conduct emergency evaluations should there be an acute change in the mental or physical health of the president or vice-president.

6. The evaluations should be strictly confidential unless the panel determines that the mental health or medical condition of the president, vice-president, or candidate renders him/her incapable of fulfilling the duties of office.

Congress must act immediately. The nuclear arsenal cannot be placed in the hands of a candidate who shows symptoms of serious mental instability. This is an urgent matter of national security. We call on our elected officials to heed the warnings of thousands of mental health professionals who have requested an independent, impartial neuropsychiatric evaluation of Mr. Trump (Greene, 2016; Lee, 2019; Phillips, 2024). The world as we know it could cease to exist with a 3 A.M. nuclear post.

Nanette Gartrell, M.D., is a psychiatrist, researcher, and writer who was formerly on the faculties of Harvard Medical School and University of California, San Francisco. Her 53 years of scientific investigations have focused primarily on sexual minority parent families. In the 1980's and '90s, Dr. Gartrell was the principal investigator of groundbreaking investigations into sexual misconduct by physicians that led to a clean-up of professional ethics codes and the criminalization of boundary violations. The Nanette K. Gartrell Papers *are archived at the Sophia Smith Collection, Smith College.*

Dee Mosbacher, M.D., Ph.D., is a psychiatrist and Academy Award-nominated documentary filmmaker who was formerly on the faculty of University of California, San Francisco. As a public-sector psychiatrist, Dr. Mosbacher specialized in the treatment of patients with severe mental illness. She served as San Mateo County's Medical Director for Mental Health and Senior Psychiatrist at San Francisco's Progress Foundation. The Diane (Dee) Mosbacher and Woman Vision Papers *are archived at the Sophia Smith Collection, Smith College. Dr. Mosbacher's films are also contained within the Smithsonian National Museum of American History collection.*

References

Abrams, H. L. (1999). Can the twenty-fifth amendment deal with a disabled president? Preventing future white house cover-ups. *Presidential Studies Quarterly* 29:115-133.

Barbaro, M. (2016, Sept 16). Donald Trump clung to "birther" lie for years, and still isn't apologetic. *The New York* Times. Retrieved from https://www.nytimes.

com/2016/09/17/us/politics/donald-trump-obama-birther.html?_r=1

Berisha, V., Wang, S., LaCross, A. & Liss, J. (2015): Tracking discourse complexity preceding Alzheimer's disease diagnosis: A case study comparing the press conferences of presidents Ronald Reagan and George Herbert Walker Bush. *Journal of Alzheimer's Disease* 45:959-963.

Carter, J. (1994). Presidential disability and the twenty-fifth amendment: A president's perspective." *JAMA* 272:1698.

Colón-Francia, A., & Fortner, J. (2014, February 27). Air Force improves its personnel reliability program. *U.S. Air Force News*. Retrieved from http://www.af.mil/News/Article-Display/Article/473435/af-improves-its-personnel-reliability-program/

Cornell University Law School. (2017). U.S. constitution 25th amendment. Retrieved from https://www.law.cornell.edu/constitution/amendmentxxv

Davidson, J. R.T., Connor, K. M., & Swartz, M. (2006). Mental illness in U.S. presidents between 1776 and 1974: A review of biographical sources. *Journal of Nervous and Mental Disease* 194:47-51.

DelReal, J. A., & Gearan, A. (2016, July 30). Trump stirs outrage after he lashes out at the Muslim parents of a dead U.S. soldier. *The Washington Post*. Retrieved from https://www.washingtonpost.com/politics/backlash-for-trump-after-he-lashes-out-at-the-muslim-parents-of-a-dead-us-soldier/2016/07/30/34b0aad4-5671-11e6-88eb-7dda4e2f2aec_story.html?utm_term=.b5ffdee05a40

Glaister, D. (2008, December 3). Recordings reveal Richard Nixon's paranoia. *The Guardian*. Retrieved from https://www.theguardian.com/world/2008/dec/03/richard-nixon-tapes

Goodwin, R. N. (1988, August 21). President Lyndon Johnson: The war within. *The New York Times*. *Retrieved from* http://www.nytimes.com/1988/08/21/magazine/president-lyndon-johnson-the-war-within.html?pagewanted=all

Greene, R. (2016, December 17). Is Donald Trump mentally ill? 3 professors of psychiatry ask President Obama to conduct "a full medical and neuropsychiatric evaluation." *Huffington Post*. Retrieved from http://www.huffingtonpost.com/richard-greene/is-donald-trump-mentally_b_13693174.html

Kendall, B. (2016, June 3). Trump says judge's Mexican heritage presents "absolute conflict." *The Wall Street Journal*. Retrieved from https://www.wsj.com/articles/donald-trump-keeps-up-attacks-on-judge-gonzalo-curiel-1464911442

Lee, B. X. (Ed.) (2019). *The Dangerous Case of Donald Trump: 37 Psychiatrists and*

Mental Health Experts Assess a President-updated and expanded with new essays. Thomas Dunne Books.

Miller, G., & Jaffe, G. (2017, May 15). Trump revealed highly classified information to Russian foreign minister and ambassador. *The Washington Post. Retrieved from* https://www.washingtonpost.com/world/national-security/trump-revealed-highly-classified-information-to-russian-foreign-minister-and-ambassador/2017/05/15/530c172a-3960-11e7-9e48-c4f199710b69_story.html?utm_term=.495bc0f95d9d

Montanaro, D. (2024, August 11). 162 lies and distortions in a news conference. NPR fact-checks former President Trump *NPR.* Retrieved from https://www.npr.org/2024/08/11/nx-s1-5070566/trump-news-conference

Osnos, E. (2017, May 1). How Trump could get fired. *The New Yorke.* Retrieved from http://www.newyorker.com/magazine/2017/05/08/how-trump-could-get-fired

Pelosi, N. (2024). *The art of power: My story as America's first woman speaker of the house.* Simon and Schuster.

Phillips, A. (2024, March 20). Donald Trump dementia evidence "overwhelming," says top psychiatrist. *Newsweek.*

Reilly, K. (2016, August 31). Here are all the times Donald Trump insulted Mexico. *Time.* Retrieved from http://time.com/4473972/donald-trump-mexico-meeting-insult/

Sebastian, M. (2016, March 15). Here's how presidents and candidates who aren't Donald Trump respond to protesters. *Esquire.* Retrieved from http://www.esquire.com/news-politics/news/a43020/heres-how-presidents-and-candidates-who-arent-donald-trump-respond-to-protesters/

TIME Staff. (2024, April 30). Read the full transcripts of Donald Trump's interviews with TIME. *TIME Retrieved from*
https://time.com/6972022/donald-trump-transcript-2024-election/

Wagner, A. (2017, February 17). Trump vs. the very fake news media. *The Atlantic. Retrieved from* https://www.theatlantic.com/politics/archive/2017/02/trump-vs-the-very-fake-news-media/516561/

Weinstein, E. A. (1981). *Woodrow Wilson: A medical and psychological biography.* Princeton, NJ: Princeton University Press.

Zaru, D. (2017, March 7). It took FOIA for park service to release photos of Obama, Trump inauguration crowd sizes. *CNN Politics.* Retrieved from http://www.cnn.com/2017/03/07/politics/national-park-service-inauguration-crowd-size-photos/

THE MYTH OF TRUMP IS A SYMPTOM OF A DEEPER PATHOLOGY

Ian Hughes, Ph.D.

The philosopher Walter Benjamin, reflecting on the rise of fascism in Europe in the 1930s, wrote of the Angel of History, whose wings were caught by the winds of progress. This wind was propelling it inexorably into the future to which its back was turned, allowing it only to watch helplessly as the wreckage of so-called "civilization" piled ever higher at its feet (Benjamin, 2020).

Today, the winds of progress have turned once again into a gale which is blowing us ever faster towards destruction. Images of war in Ukraine, an unending spiral of violence in the Middle East, rising tensions with China, the willful destruction of democracy in the United States, and the re-emergence of the far right across Europe, assail us every day.

The term that has been coined to describe this confluence of dangerous events is "polycrisis". It is meant to not only denote simply the fact that multiple crises are occurring simultaneously, but also to warn that each individual crisis—if not dealt with successfully—will likely exacerbate and accelerate all of the others.

Within this threatening and volatile context, two 'events' stand out as exceptional in their potential to act as accelerants of our potential destruction—climate change and the re-election of Donald Trump.

Floods, heat waves, hurricanes, and wildfires are becoming ever more frequent and intense. Even the richest countries are not prepared to cope with these rapidly worsening impacts of climate change. Poorer countries are already facing the realities of mass emigration and economic collapse as food systems fail, lands become inundated or desertified, and temperatures rise to levels that make human habitation impossible. Scientists warn that these accelerating impacts are now pushing our planetary systems into dangerous instability.

In this maelstrom, the re-election of Donald Trump as President of the United States, if it were to happen, would likely exacerbate all of the individual crises the world is facing—a further erosion of democracy in the United States, a strengthening of the alliance of authoritarian strongmen across the globe, a sharp increase in tensions with China, a victory for Putin in Ukraine, and a further loss of hope for peace in the Middle East. It would also mark the return of vociferous climate denial, just at the moment when delayed action will push the world towards unavoidable climate disaster.

Where lies Hope?

In Irish poet Seamus Heaney's poem 'From the Canton of Expectation', he writes of the profound consequences of education becoming available en masse to those whose destiny had been to suffer injustice. All over the world people are struggling to understand the causes and solutions to these crises. Writers are using their pens to dig for deeper truths to explain our current situation; activists are using their feet—and giving their lives—to create a better future; artists are rousing within us our innate longing for justice. As a result, "intelligences brightened and unmannerly as crow bars", as Heaney wrote, are allowing us to begin to see the true roots of our dysfunction.

As a result, two profound truths are becoming clear.

First, the roots of the contemporary polycrisis lie deep within both our psychology and the template of our civilization.

Donald Trump's election as President in 2016 was a profound shock to many within the United States and around the world. At that time, much of the analysis focused on Trump as a toxic personality and the threat he posed as an individual to America's democratic system (Lee, 2019). The discussion today has changed in two important ways. First, while Trump's pathological character remains a focus, he is no longer seen as a solitary figure, but instead as one of a large number of so-called 'strongman' leaders. In the last decades, a series of such leaders has emerged within both democracies and authoritarian states. Besides Trump, the list includes Vladimir Putin in Russia, Xi Jinping in China, Mohammed bin Salman in Saudi Arabia, Narendra Modi in India, Jair Bolsonaro in Brazil, Recep Tayyep Erdogan in Turkey, and Viktor Orbán in Hungary. Taken together, our era of the 'Strongman leader' can be seen to be one of the defining features of early twenty-first century geopolitics (Rachman, 2022). This phenomenon is, of course, not new, but also characterized much of the twentieth century, the century of

Hitler, Stalin, Mao, and many, many other pathological tyrants (Hughes, 2018).

The problem of Trump can therefore be restated within a broader global and historical context. The conditions which give rise to Trump-style fascism occur frequently, and when they do, there is something in our psychology that prompts large sections of the population to empower pathological leaders and support their oppressive and violent agendas.

The recognition that he is part of a recurring systemic global phenomenon has led to a second change in the discourse on Trump this time around. It has prompted an examination of the systems that are empowering not only him but all his fellow authoritarians around the world. The explanation that is emerging, both for Trump and for authoritarianism in general, lies both in individual psychopathology and in our dysfunctional social systems.

Let us consider first those dysfunctional systems, namely our political, economic, and cultural systems. Philosopher Alain Badiou (2022) has highlighted that these systems are predominantly hierarchical in nature, and are based upon what Raine Eisler and Douglas Fry have termed dominance values (Eisler & Fry, 2019). Dominance values include rigid top-down rankings, the acceptance of gross inequalities, hyper-masculinity and the denigration of women, hyper-competition, cultural acceptance of abuse and violence, and use of fear and force to preserve the structural violence that is embedded within the system. Our contemporary economic, political, and cultural systems are all, to one degree or another, dominance systems.

One crucial feature of these systems is that they empower individuals who hold matching dominance values, enabling them to thrive and rise to power within those systems. And of course, the human beings who excel, par excellence, in dominance values are the types of dangerous individuals that the authors of this volume are highlighting, namely psychopaths and those who suffer from personality disorders such as narcissistic personality disorder, paranoid personality disorder and malignant narcissism (Wood, 2022). The types of individuals who thrive best within dominance systems are persons who feel no empathy for others, who view others as objects to be used or threats to be eliminated, and for whom the concept of equality is impossible to conceive. Research in psychology shows clearly that there is a sizeable number of such individuals in every society on earth. The disturbing fact is that the design of most of our social institutions empowers them to take control over the rest of us.

A second profound truth is also becoming clearer: Alongside these hierarchical dominance systems, with their values of violence, racism, sexism, and homophobia, lies a parallel system based on egalitarian values and social practices which reject violence and support equality, compassion, caring and cooperation. This system of social networks, based on altruism, empathy, and gift exchange, is always present and became radically visible in many places during the Covid pandemic, for example. A more humane template for our societies already exists.

The challenge for this generation is to disempower the hierarchical dominance systems, with their male narcissistic leaders, and empower instead the empathic networks which value the sacred ordinary of relationships, beauty, empathy, equality, love, and fun.

Much of the current discourse on the changes we need to make to address the polycrisis of climate change, political dysfunction, destabilizing inequalities, and far right fascism focus on technology and economic growth as remedies. The problems, however, are much more complex, as are the social systems we need to reform to address those problems. The problems run deeper and so too must be the solutions we seek.

Systems thinking tells us that while solutions to complex problems are usually sought at the level of practical everyday interventions, the greatest leverage for fundamental change comes from changing our mental models of the world. And within our mental models of the world, myth plays an essential role. Unfortunately, many myths we currently live by are having enormously destructive impacts on our relationships with one another and with Nature.

In economics, the myth of Homo economicus holds that human beings are rational and narrowly self-interested agents. This myth denigrates and devalorizes the other, more fundamental, economies upon which society is based—the gift society of moral, reciprocal, altruistic exchange (Mauss, 2016), and the emotional economy whereby our relationships with others are governed by feelings owed or owing (Hochschild, 2002).

Much of global politics is based on the twin myths of the primacy of hypermasculinity, and the myth of redemptive violence. The first tells us that only strong men who exhibit traits of dominance, narcissism, aggression and competitiveness are fit for leadership. The myth of redemptive violence tells us that violence will solve our problems, that war and genocide will somehow bring peace and security.

In technology, we are increasingly being forced to live by the myth of creative destruction, that technologies, developed and diffused throughout society by a small number of hyper-wealthy and powerful individuals, regardless of their socially destructive impacts, is what counts as progress.

Gender is still largely shaped by the myth of binary genders, that empathy, love, care, fragility, need, and vulnerability are signs of "feminine' weakness, rather than the relational means through which all human beings develop and form the conditions necessary for our continued flourishing.

In religion, the myth of a knowable, violent, hypermasculine god who wills inequalities and oppression, survives alongside a broader mythology that sees the sacred as an unknowable source of Nature's wonder and human existence and love.

It is upon these destructive myths that infuse our mental models of the world that violent narcissistic leaders rise to power.

Trump and the far right have an impoverished view of humanity and a fear-filled view of the world. They would force us all to live on a smaller stage, so small that they need to expel or eliminate anyone who doesn't think and look like them. In the face of the challenges that the future is presenting us with, we need to live on a much larger stage and embrace a more inclusive and expansive view of humanity and a much richer vision for the future of our societies.

Disordered minds like Donald Trump are psychologically incapable of either living within inclusive presents or forging pathways to expansive futures. *The myth of Trump is that he is a promise that will never materialize—a promise to fix complex problems on the basis of narcissism, hatred and fear.*

The lesson that Trump is offering us is that the end of our current civilization is something we should welcome and work towards. A new civilization based on foundational myths that allow us to flourish rather than fight is what this generation must strive towards. Myths that allow us to love the diversity of humanity and care for the only planet on which we know for sure that the miracle of life exists. The Angel of History is blown into the future by the stories we tell and the myths we embrace. When these stories change, old civilizations fall and new ones rise to meet the future. If we are to embrace that future, we must reject the myth of Trump and urgently reimagine a new and more radical way forward.

Ian Hughes, Ph.D., is a scientist and author. He has a doctorate in experimental atomic physics from Queen's University in Belfast, and a Postgraduate Diploma in Psychoanalytic Psychotherapy from the Irish Institute for Psychoanalytic Psychotherapy, which has informed his work. He is a

Senior Research Fellow at the MaREI Centre, Environmental Research Institute, University College Cork, Ireland. His book, Disordered Minds: How Dangerous Personalities Are Destroying Democracy, *explores how a small proportion of people with dangerous personality disorders are responsible for most of the violence and greed that disfigures our world.*

References

Badiou, A. (2022). *A new dawn for politics*. John Wiley & Sons.

Benjamin, W. (2020). *Theses on the philosophy of history. In critical theory and society* (pp. 255-263). Routledge.

Eisler, R., & Fry, D. P. (2019). *Nurturing our humanity: How domination and partnership shape our brains, lives, and future.* Oxford University Press.

Hochschild, A. R. (2002). *The sociology of emotion as a way of seeing.* In *emotions in social life*. Routledge.

Hughes, I. (2018). *Disordered minds: How dangerous personalities are destroying democracy*, Zero Books.

Lee, B. X. (2019). *The dangerous case of Donald Trump: 37 psychiatrists and mental health experts assess a president-updated and expanded with new essays*. Thomas Dunne Books.

Mauss, M. (2016). *The Gift*. Jane I. Guyer (Expanded ed.). Chicago.

Rachman, G. (2022). *The age of the strongman: How the cult of the leader threatens democracy around the world*. Random House.

Wood, R. (2022). *A study of malignant narcissism: Personal and professional insights*. Routledge.

Printed in Great Britain
by Amazon

59850299R00145